Rebuilding Health

Rebuilding Health

The Waerland Method of Natural Therapy
with Case History

by

Ebba Waerland

Translated by Isabella M. Gibbs
Introduction by Douglas Latto, M.B., Ch.B.

The Lutterworth Press
Cambridge

Published by
The Lutterworth Press
P.O. Box 60
Cambridge
CB1 2NT
England

e-mail: **publishing@lutterworth.com**
website: **http://www.lutterworth.com**

ISBN 0 7188 9130 9 hardback
ISBN 0 7188 9129 5 paperback

British Library Cataloguing in Publication Data:
A catalogue record is available from the British Library.

First published by James Clarke & Co, 1966,
reprinted 2002

Contents

Introduction by Dr. Douglas Latto
Foreword by A. V. Knack / xi
About the author / xiii
Introduction / xvii
1 / *Building and maintaining health / 3*
2 / *Seven golden rules for health / 13*
3 / *Daily program for health / 15*
4 / *How to make the change / 22*
5 / *My own case history / 31*
6 / *The physiologically correct fast / 43*
7 / *Rheumatism, gout, and arthritis / 47*
8 / *Asthma / 59*
9 / *Cancer / 67*
10 / *Diabetes / 78*
11 / *Eczema and psoriasis / 91*
12 / *Diseases of the stomach and intestines; ulcers / 98*
13 / *Diseases of the liver, kidneys, and gall bladder / 114*
14 / *Multiple sclerosis / 127*
15 / *Dropsy / 136*
16 / *Tuberculosis of the lungs / 142*
17 / *Headache, migraine, insomnia, and constipation / 151*
18 / *Anemia, high blood pressure, heart disorders / 160*
19 / *Goitre / 172*
20 / *Varicose veins, leg ulcers, abscesses, sinusitis / 180*
21 / *The value of correct breathing / 189*
22 / *Conclusion: the mental and spiritual / 192*
23 / *Recipes and instructions / 195*
24 / *Nature's rich dispensary: herbs / 210*
Glossary / 241
Index / 247

Introduction

by Douglas Latto, M.B., Ch.B.

I have read from cover to cover this most refreshing and vital book.

It is obvious that Mrs. Ebba Waerland has regained a state of real positive health.

When working in Oxford I met the famous nutritionist, Sir Robert McCarrison, on several occasions. He always said to me that the three necessities he demanded of food were:

1. It should be grown on healthy soil.
2. It should be eaten whole.
3. It should be eaten fresh.

I would like to illustrate these three essential requirements:

1. It is important that the soil in which we grow our food is healthy. The mass medication of the soil with seed 'dressings', artificial fertilizers, selective weed killers, pesticides, etc., do not make for healthy soil and, therefore, the plants are unhealthy.
2. The food should be eaten whole, that is as nature intended us to eat it. If one takes a grain of wheat and breaks it down into its component parts: white flour, bran, vitamins, mineral salts, etc., and then tries to put it together again something invariably gets lost or out of balance.

We can all take a daisy apart and examine it in detail, but none of us can put it together again.

3. The food should be eaten soon after it has been taken from the soil. It is then at its highest potential. If it is kept for a time the vitamins begin to disappear, some faster than others. If it is preserved by canning, heating, freezing, etc., it also drops in potential.

The above three simple requirements have been well underlined by Ebba Waerland in this book.

It should be read by all doctors and would give a new impetus to preventive medicine.

Foreword

by A. V. Knack, Prof. Med.

[*Dr. Knack, a leader of the official medical service of Hamburg, Germany, was medical director of the official clinic, Barmbeck, of that city, and later was president of the official health magistracy there. He was a leader in health-reform movements in Europe.*]

I have decided after mature deliberation to write a few introductory lines to this book, because I am anxious for doctors as well as laymen to read and concern themselves with the very interesting experiences of this well-known writer, which I consider most valuable on account of their great objectivity.

For the first time a comprehensive and detailed description of the Waerland system of treating disease is presented with supporting case histories to illustrate it. At the same time its publication should be safe from superficial criticism by the wealth of material proving its efficacy.

The author has been exceedingly ingenious in her skillful adaptation of the fundamental food reforms worked out by Are Waerland in the sphere of dietetic treatment of disease. In doing so she has by no means taken a one-sided attitude but has included other already-tested natural methods of treatment.

Her own remarkable experience has made her an inspired and enthusiastic advocate of these ideas, and the whole book bears witness to this enthusiasm. It will be the task of science to test what she has presented. As a physician of wide experience I am convinced that the verdict will be favorable. In this belief I wish Ebba Waerland's book every success and wide distribution.

About the author

Ebba Waerland was born Ebba Margareta Langenskiöld on October 15, 1897, in Stockholm, Sweden, of Finnish ancestry on both sides. In 1922 she married Eduard Hoffman, a German diplomat, and had two children. Her husband died in 1940.

In 1946 she married the famous nutritional physiologist, writer, and philosopher, Are Waerland. Dr. Waerland, who graduated from the University of Helsingfors and did post-graduate work at Uppsala, Paris, London, and Edinburgh, was the founder of the reformed diet and way of life which bears his name and now extends to the far corners of the earth. Sanatoriums based on his principles are found in Germany, Sweden, Switzerland, Italy, and Iceland, and the Waerland diet is available in hotels and boarding-houses in many countries. A Waerland department is planned for a government hospital in Syria.

Ebba Waerland became Dr. Waerland's closest co-worker. She founded and directed Kiholm, the first Swedish sanatorium practicing the Waerland principles, and later a number in other countries. She trained physicians in these methods and developed the famous Waerland diet adaptations and therapies. A speaker of seven languages, she has carried on lecture tours in various countries and is associated with many health-reform magazines.

Ebba Waerland was active in both world wars. At eighteen, she helped to recruit the Swedish brigade that aided the Finns against the invading Russians in the first war. During the second, she made her home a place of refuge for Finnish refugees, taking in forty mothers and their children. She smuggled food and clothing to Finnish relief organizations. After the collapse of Germany, she started and financed the first large relief undertaking to ease the condition of refugees from the east.

For several decades she aided the social work of churches among liberated prisoners, the unemployed, and the homeless. Her aim through life has been to mitigate physical and spiritual distress and to assist people and enterprises that work for the betterment of mankind. Her second husband, Are Waerland, died in 1955, at seventy-nine.

Mrs. Waerland is the author of many books. Her first book of poetry was published in 1918, when she was twenty. Other works are six collections of poems, two translations of German and Italian lyrics, eight ethical religious books, three story books, numerous books and pamphlets on diet and way of life, a philosophical work, a book and two pamphlets on the dangers of nuclear reactions in peace and war. Also she has translated ten books and fifteen pamphlets by Are Waerland.

Because Mrs. Waerland's results with her patients have been so spectacularly successful, her American publisher wrote her a discreet letter as the book was about to go to press inquiring about possible failures. The correspondence follows:

Dear Mrs. Waerland:
Your manuscript is now ready for the printer. May I again tell you how profoundly impressed we are by it.

One question. While your case histories are entirely convincing I cannot help wondering about the failures. Surely you must have had them, especially with those individuals who had no innate will to live. I believe a paragraph or two citing some of these and perhaps mentioning the proportion of failures to sucesses would be in order.

DEVIN A. GARRITY

Dear Mr. Garrity:

You ask me to give a paragraph or two on my "failures." I am sorry, but I don't remember any failures. Often I have had patients for a very short time—seven to ten days or a fortnight—and naturally I can't obtain real healings in such a short time. But I have always noticed that the patient has made progress in some way. At least the patient has understood better the ways and means of building up new health, and he has had more confidence in the possibility of recovery. In most cases he has had new hope and a new, positive feeling toward life.

Also, I very often have had patients who were hopelessly ill. Their physicians had said that they had only a few weeks more of life. In desperation, they have come to me as a last resort. I tell them that I don't know if I can help them, but "where there is life there is hope."

It is wonderful to feel the confidence they have in me. This feeling of trust and security gives great relief to those patients who cannot be saved. But in several cases I have witnessed a miracle, as the natural healing forces in a body on the threshold of another life again have won the struggle with the forces of destruction—and the patient has recovered.

EBBA WAERLAND

Introduction

Some years ago I was delivered from untold suffering, which I had endured since childhood, through adopting the way of living we now refer to as the Waerland System.

Ever since then I have felt that my vocation was to try to help as many other sufferers as possible.

The joy of returning to life after so many years of pain, having fought against discouragement and having finally abandoned all hope of recovery, gave me a tremendous urge to share my happiness with others and lead them on the road to health as I had been led.

In my school of suffering and especially in finding my way back to normal life, I learned much that now stands me in good stead in my new calling as adviser and guide to thousands of sick people. For we can only truly understand the things we ourselves have experienced.

This book has been written at the request of a great many people in various parts of the world, and I am very happy to comply with their wishes. I have endeavored to describe in simple terms the natural, biological methods which have been tested and have given good results in treating all kinds of diseases. I have described a number of cases successfully treated by these methods, many of which had been given up by doctors.

My methods are, of course, based on the work of Are Waerland, my late husband, who spent the greater part of his life in research and experiment on the problem of health and disease and, through his prolific writing, pointed out the way of health in a rapidly declining civilization.*

I have always been very happy to be permitted to collaborate with members of the medical profession, in cases when they made the diagnosis and followed the progress of the treatment, to our mutual help and advantage. I am especially glad to have this opportunity of thanking Dr. Östling, who so courageously supported our work at Kiholm (Sweden) and, in fact, made it possible for us to carry on our activities there.

It is my earnest wish that this book may be the means of helping many suffering men and women to free themselves from their disorders and find their way back to health.

EBBA WAERLAND

Skärvik, Djursholm, Sweden

* As, for example, *In the Cauldron of Disease,* Are Waerland's first major book on the subject. Published by David Nutt, London, 1934. (Out of print.)

Rebuilding health:

THE WAERLAND METHOD OF NATURAL THERAPY

1 / Building and maintaining health

The last twenty years have seen a fundamental change in our view of health and disease. Scientific discoveries in the fields of nutrition, chemistry, and biology have shown that what we have come to call "diseases of civilization" are largely self-incurred and that their source can be traced to a faulty diet and other mistakes in the way we arrange our lives.

Much of this was realized more than forty years ago by Are Waerland, whose teaching has since brought new life and health to thousands of people.

The basic maxim behind all Waerland's work—the result of a lifetime of research and experiment—is the bold declaration: *"We are not concerned with diseases but with MISTAKES IN LIVING. Get rid of the mistakes and the diseases will disappear of their own accord."*

How do we begin?

First and foremost by adopting a diet which leaves behind the least possible amount of harmful residues in the body and does not cause putrefaction in the intestines, thereby poisoning the whole system.

We begin then by cutting out meat, fish, and eggs from

our daily meals, since, during the process of digestion, these foods—even when cooked—provide a fertile culture medium for putrefactive microbes which, owing to the great length of the human digestive tract, are capable of producing large quantities of toxic matter in the body. The diseases of civilization are partly toxic and partly deficiency diseases caused by unnatural, disease-producing foods and a way of life that is unsuited to our physiological make-up.

Professor Wilska, of the University of Helsingfors, has demonstrated that, by exposure to heat, poisons are produced in all foods containing animal protein and cholesterol. He calls these poisons "mortamins" and has already discovered three hundred different species of them in meat, fish, cheese, and even in heated milk and in butter. This disposes of the theory that the cooking of animal protein foods protects us from their injurious effects.

A lacto-vegetarian raw diet, i.e., a diet consisting of raw green and root vegetables, cereals—whole and unadulterated—milk and milk products, fulfills all the requirements for building a healthy body. It is only through living food, rich in vitamins, auxones,* minerals, trace elements and alkaline salts, that the living body is able to build healthy, vigorous cells.

Research by the well-known scientist Dr. Rusch has demonstrated that the eating of cooked foods sets up a digestive leucocytosis in the intestinal tract which, in the long run, becomes dangerous to health.

Our digestive system has a most ingenious signaling ar-

* See Glossary.

rangement: as soon as unnatural food is put into the mouth, "danger signals" are sent to the intestinal tract. If the food we are eating has been cooked or treated in any way that robs it of vitality or splits it into micro-parts, the independently working filtering process in the walls of the intestines is no longer able to protect the body against an invasion of foreign substances through the mucous membrane. To prevent these substances from penetrating into the blood and tissues, the alarm is given to the white corpuscles, the leucocytes, which are able to absorb foreign micro-organisms and render them harmless. At the danger signal the mucous membranes are flooded with leucocytes. But repeated calling into action of this kind of protective guard, intended as an emergency measure, weakens and deranges the functioning of the body, thereby lessening its resistance.

Rawkost* (a diet of mainly raw foods), on the other hand, does not produce this leucocytosis, and even if a meal is begun with something raw in the form of a salad and then a small quantity of cooked food follows, no harm is done; but the raw food should always predominate on the menu.

These facts are surely sufficient to show that our digestive apparatus was originally developed for the purpose of digesting living foods from the vegetable kingdom. Other evidence of this is the natural bacterial flora of the intestines. The intestinal tract of a healthy child is populated by the type of bacteria required to break down cellulose. It is only when the child is given meat, fish, or eggs

* See glossary.

that the flora is changed and the putrefactive bacteria begin to predominate. This is the beginning of the ever-increasing poisoning of civilized man and the organic decay which is manifested in innumerable diseases.

Animal protein is not the only culprit to be blamed for the dangers of our civilized diet. In these days almost all foods are refined, denatured, and robbed of their most valuable qualities. We have only to consider white sugar, which has had all its living substances removed. Sugar cane is a complete food containing a percentage of sugar which suits our body. Refined sugar, on the other hand, drains our system of vitally important substances: minerals, vitamins, and calcium. We cannot assimilate it in its unnaturally concentrated form without drawing on our own supplies of elements which are indispensable for the maintenance of our cells.

Ordinary commercial salt, used for cooking and on the table, bottles up unhealthy fluids in the tissues and is one of the main causes of rheumatism. Living vegetable foods contain ample supplies of sodium chloride and other alkaline salts, and every addition of inorganic salt is harmful.

Another source of poisoning in our foods is the use of artificial preservatives and coloring matter. Medical authorities are warning the public more and more against these chemicals, which may be direct causes of cancer.

Strong spices and condiments irritate the mucous membranes of the digestive tract. Tea, coffee, and cocoa contain certain injurious drugs and slowly undermine our health. The nicotine in tobacco poisons not only the smoker himself but all those around him. When tobacco is burned, certain cancer-causing tar substances are formed. Cancer of the lungs is finding many of its victims among women, since so many women now smoke. Statistics have shown a definite connection between cancer of the lungs and tobacco smoking.

Overcooked food and refined white flour lead to constipation. The colon becomes slack and distended and the rectum is turned into a breeding ground for all kinds of infections. Our great detoxicating organ, the liver, becomes overloaded and breaks down. The organs of elimination are no longer able to rid us of all the poisons which are daily and hourly introduced into our bodies in the form of foods and drinks, stimulants and narcotics.

What, then, does civilized man do in his despair? Instead of trying to build up new cells by means of a diet that will give the body all the elements of sound nutrition, he flies to injurious drug treatments and unnatural means of disguising the symptoms without going to the root cause of the trouble. In this way he slides further and further into the mire.

The great Greek physician, the father of medicine, Hippocrates, said, "Your medicine shall be your food and your food your medicine." Modern experience in the physiology of nutrition has proved how right he was. In complete living foods, i.e., those containing all the essentials of nutrition, we have all the elements required for building up health. Take, for instance, the green leaf, with its wealth of chlorophyll. It was American doctors who first discovered the marvelous effect of chlorophyll in treating septic diseases. Remarkable results in healing were achieved through injections of chlorophyll even in the most severe cases, and it was not long before it was introduced into European hospitals.

The question then arises: why lower the resistance of the body through the deficiency of organic, health-building foods in the diet, only to resort to synthetically produced preparations to repair the damage? Would it not be more reasonable and practical to *start* with a physiologically correct dietary which would build robust cells and give *natural* immunity to disease?

The truth of Hippocrates' thesis, that it is by healthful food that a healthy body can be built up, has been amply proved during the past twenty years by thousands of sick people in various countries who have regained their health by adopting the Waerland diet.

The health of the soil

But we cannot win back perfect health unless the plants and products of nature that go to make up our food are themselves organically sound, containing all the vital elements that make them complete. And here we find yet another way in which civilization has frustrated its own ends and by wrong treatment has impoverished and poisoned the soil. We force the soil to produce large crops and then use unnatural means to restore the constituents it loses in the process. Even in the soil the balance of metabolism is achieved, and if this balance is upset, deficiencies and pathological changes take place. The micro-organisms essential for all healthy vegetation cannot flourish in artificially fertilized soil, since chemically produced fertilizer is as unsuitable for the soil as our chemically treated food is for the human body. When the micro-organisms and the earthworms disappear, the soil becomes sterile and eventually eroded.

The unadulterated products of the good earth build up our health. But it is not only good food that we need. Pure drinking water from wells that are not befouled by sewage —a drink that does not need disinfecting with poisonous chemicals—is equally important.

Milk

We also need milk and milk products from healthy cows. If our domestic animals are allowed to live according to the laws of nature, they will be healthy and the need to vitiate milk by sterilization will no longer exist.

Air

Our present-day superficial and very limited hygiene is not capable of keeping diseases away. To create the inward cleanliness that is essential for true health, we must go to war against everything that sullies the mainsprings of our life. The chief of these is the air. Life entails combustion, and for all the life processes of our organism we need oxygen. We need pure air, free from poisonous gases and fumes. This is very difficult to find in our civilized communities where exhaust fumes, chimney smoke, and vapors from chemical factories pollute the atmosphere. Not many of us are privileged to live in ozone-filled air, away from the impurities of cities and towns.

All the functions of the body are conditioned by their surroundings. Let us restore to our organs their original, natural life element, and they will regain their lost life rhythm. Wonderful results have already shown what can be done with a way of life based on this principle, that is, by restoring to our organs their true functional components: to our digestive organs complete and living foods, to our lungs pure air and, not least, the releasing of our skin from the prison of heavy, closely woven clothing so that it may react to fresh air, sunlight, cold water, and changes of temperature. Only through "toughening" in these ways will our resistance be increased and the skin, an enormous breathing and detoxicating organ, function at its best. By vigorous brushing and reasonable care, we must keep it supple and elastic.

All our excretory organs are dependent upon a sufficient intake of fluids. We must drink plentifully between meals in order to get rid of all the residual substances, or "dregs," which otherwise will be piled up in our organism during the processes of digestion and metabolism. If the organs of elimination do not function fully, the poisons will be left behind to create auto-intoxication in the body; our health will then deteriorate and disease will follow.

The strenuous intensity of modern life puts a tremendous strain upon our nerves. Many of us lead a sedentary life with insufficient exercise in the fresh air, and this leads to the slow wasting of the muscles and accumulation of residues in the body, owing to sluggish circulation of the blood. On the other hand, our nervous energy is often sapped by a hectic life rhythm and a whirl of excitement and sensation. The proper balance between physical activity and discipline on the one hand, and a calm, collected and tranquil mind on the other, has been upset. The consequences are to be seen in the alarming increase in nervous diseases.

Health is, however, not governed merely by physical processes. A human being is an inseparable unity consisting of body, mind, and spirit. Scientists are devoting increasing attention to the part played by psychological influences in health and disease. In a recent German medical journal, Dr. Rink described experiments carried out by an American professor, Dr. Harrison Bean, showing the influence our attitude to life, our moods, and our reactions to outward circumstances exert on our physical well-being. The professor has discovered a method of condensing people's breath and of registering the different colorings of the condensations. When the condensed breath was injected into animals, it produced the most varied effects. In many cases the animals did not react at all; in other cases the reaction was violent, with symptoms pointing to acute poisoning. One of the animals died after being injected with the breath of a man who was filled with hate.

All negative emotions such as hate and anger, distress and deep melancholy create poisonous secretions in the glands of the body. It has, for instance, long been known that the venom of a cobra is far more poisonous when the creature is excited.

Just as negative reactions and emotions have a destructive effect, a positive attitude to life releases reserves of energy and vitality that are practically unlimited.

Only by ordering our lives in harmony with the laws of nature are we able to build up true health. This we can do by introducing into our daily living the positive health-building life factors reviewed here, and by turning away from the disease-producing habits and ingrained prejudices of so-called civilized living.

2 / *Seven golden rules for health*

1. *Build up healthy, vigorous cells by giving your body foods that will supply all its needs,* i.e., lacto-vegetarian rawkost* (raw vegetables, whole cereals, and milk products).
2. *Do not destroy your green and root vegetables by cooking them.* Heat changes or destroys the mineral substances and vitamins, also half of the organic nutriment, a third to four fifths of the sugar, a sixth to four fifths of the starch, and one fifth to one half of the protein.
3. *Assist the work of all the organs of elimination by giving the body plenty of fluids.* As the body excretes from five to six pints of fluids daily, this quantity must be compensated for. A normal lacto-vegetarian diet provides in the daily food about three pints of fluids. The rest should be taken in liquid form, between meals during the course of the day.
4. *Take care that the waste products are adequately removed from the body by the organs of elimination,* mainly, that is, by the great bowel, in the form of two or three evacuations in the twenty-four hours, but also via the skin through perspiration, which should be induced by suitable exercise, preferably in the fresh air,

* See Glossary.

and through a Sauna* (Finnish) or other form of hot-air bath once a week (for persons with no heart weakness).

5. *Do not weaken the intestines by the continued use of enemas or laxatives.* The enema should be used only during special cleansing or fasting periods and cannot be used regularly for longer than a month at a time without seriously relaxing the muscles and damaging the mucous membranes. (Daily douches of the rectum with no more than one pint of fluid are not harmful.) No chemical laxatives should be used.
6. *Give your blood as much oxygen as possible* by sleeping with windows open and spending as much time as possible in pure fresh air, and by avoiding everything which can introduce toxins into the blood, such as tobacco fumes and bad air in close, ill-ventilated places.
7. *Cultivate a positive, cheerful attitude toward life* and learn to control your thoughts and emotions so that you are able to overcome negative, devitalizing thoughts and feelings by striving to build an inner life dominated by peace, harmony, and joy.

* See Glossary.

3 / Daily program for health

"We are not concerned with diseases but with mistakes in living. Get rid of the mistakes and the diseases will disappear of their own accord."

ARE WAERLAND

For many years Are Waerland followed and advocated the daily health program given below. It incorporates all the health-building factors evolved through his biological studies and research and has proved its validity in thousands of lives.

From this general system the particular dietetic treatments have been developed and adapted for specific diseases.

The morning drink

Begin the day immediately on waking with a good drink. Our bodies need fluid of the right kind in the early morning to help the organs of elimination to clear away poisons and residues which are products of digestion and fatigue. Much ill health is caused through the inactivity or clogging of these organs which are normally intended to keep the balance between intake and output.

Water in which potatoes and carrots have been boiled

gives a splendid supply of mineral salts and, being highly alkaline, neutralizes the acids which most people have in excess of what is normal. An excellent drink is prepared as follows: In a pint of potato (or potato-and-carrot) water, soak overnight two level tablespoonfuls of whole linseed and two of bran. Warm up slightly in the morning and drink it all, stirring to keep the linseed afloat.

Care of the skin, morning bath, and morning walk

After the drink follows a *head massage* with the finger tips, which stimulates the scalp and the activity of the brain and promotes a warm glow all over the body. Immediately afterward take either a cold bath, a cold shower, or a cold rubdown with a towel lightly wrung out in cold water, then vigorously dry with a rough towel, and scrub every inch of the body with a dry skin brush. For this, a stiff bath brush may be used, but as the skin quickly grows accustomed to the brushing, it soon begins to "ask" for a harder bristle; the Swedes often use horse-grooming brushes. When dressed we are ready for the *morning walk*. This is of the very greatest importance for the whole of the day, as it charges the blood with oxygen and tones up all the life functions—the appetite, sleep, digestion, elimination of poisons, resistance to colds and infection.

Breakfast

As the body is busy eliminating waste products up to about noon, the breakfast should be a very light meal, needing hardly any digestion, and should help in the eliminating process. For this, fruit and yogurt or, better still, homemade sour milk, to which may be added a little linseed, bran, and milk sugar, are excellent. In cold weather, potato porridge (see recipe on page 205) makes an excellent breakfast with sour milk. Dried fruits and nuts are also suitable for breakfast. All *fresh fruit* belongs to the morning and combines best with sour milk but not with sweet milk, bread, roots, or green vegetabes. Fresh fruit may also be taken between meals as the only allowable "snack." *Stewed fruit,* on the other hand, combines well with sweet or sour milk, kruska,* and potato porridge.

Lunch

If more convenient, this meal may be taken at night and the vegetable meal at midday. The best lunch for delicate stomachs is *molino** and for strong stomachs *kruska.* These dishes, with the accessories prescribed, should be taken as a meal in themselves *without any other dishes or drinks.* They contain essential food values in the balanced combination required by the body, and keep the digestion in excellent condition. The recipes will be found in the appendix.

Dinner

The basis of this meal should be a good portion of potatoes, boiled in their skins in plenty of water, without salt,

* See Glossary and Recipes.

and eaten skins and all, with finely grated raw carrots and beets. Add to this the "radium" of the vegetable kingdom, a raw onion, which should be brought *whole* to the table and cut up just before it is to be eaten, as the oxygen of the air destroys the vitamins and the flavor. (The odor of onions is neutralized almost entirely when combined as described above and with parsley.) The rest of the meal may be made up (according to circumstances of season, supplies, and purse) of lettuce, water cress, mustard greens, land cress, tomatoes, cucumbers, parsley, chives, spring onions, radishes (eat the leaves if the radishes are young), young spinach leaves, young dandelion leaves, nasturtium leaves, and any edible garden produce, as far as possible raw. If spinach is used in large quantities, it should be plunged into a large saucepan of boiling water for about ten minutes and the *water thrown away* to get rid of the oxalic acid. Serve hot with a little butter. A slice of wholemeal bread and butter with a thin slice of mild cheese and sliced onion on top makes a good complement to the vegetables. A sweet consisting of stewed fruit, or a cooked vegetable course, may be included in this meal if desired. A dish of *filbunke* (Swedish homemade sour milk) with a sprinkle of nutmeg, a little milk sugar or cane sugar, a teaspoon of grated nuts or stewed fruit, is an excellent dessert. (See recipes)

Diet adaptations

Some people find it difficult or inadvisable to make a complete change of diet suddenly. In such cases the change-over should be adapted to individual conditions. It is a good plan to begin by eliminating all the wrong things and gradually substituting the right ones.

Gastric-ulcer subjects should avoid roughage until the ulcers are well healed, proceeding very carefully on molino, potatoes, and fresh vegetable juices (diluted if too strong). Rheumatic subjects should avoid fruits, especially acid fruits and cut down on carbohydrates (bread, cereals, etc.) at first. The use of the enema is a great help to begin with in all toxic and stagnant conditions, but it should not become habitual.

Notes for health

Avoid all table salt and cooking salt (there is plenty of the right kind of salt in vegetables), also coffee, strong tea, meat, fish, eggs, drinking at meals, very hot drinks, tobacco, alcohol, sweets, chocolate, white bread, and cakes made of white flour.

Do not mix the meals. They are arranged systematically so as to complement each other and assist metabolism.

Do not add dressings, sugar, fruit, or fruit juices to salads and vegetables.

Eat live food!

In these days much food on the market is so preserved and denatured that it is worth while for good health to take some trouble to obtain fresh foods which, as far as possible, have not been tampered with. Vegetables are best home grown or obtained from growers who use organic methods. Vitamins and minerals can be seriously reduced or lost by some of the drastic chemicals used as fertilizers, sprays, and preservatives. This applies also to cereals. Compost-grown wholemeal flour, as well as other foods, can be obtained from health-food stores and from advertisers in magazines whose policies favor organic gardening and natural methods of gaining and retaining health.* Ordinary bran is best, when clean. The pasteurization of milk is at best a makeshift which, owing to present world conditions, it is difficult to remedy on a large scale as was actually done by the Finnish government some years ago, when all dairy farms were purged of diseased cattle, which were replaced by healthy ones, and the farms modernized and made hygienic under strict supervision. Fresh, unpasteurized milk is, however, obtainable in parts of the United States and, to a certain extent, in Britain, and should always be used whenever possible. Food reformers in Scandinavia have made enormous changes in supplies of live food—simply by creating a demand.

Baths

Too-frequent warm baths are not good, but once a week a warm bath is beneficial. The skin is much "cleaner" with daily friction and brushing than with numerous baths. If at first you cannot "face" a cold sponge or shower in the

* Magazines such as *Natural Food and Farming*, Atlanta, Texas; *Organic Gardening and Farming* and *Prevention*, both at Emmaus, Pa.; *Let's Live*, 133 N. Vermont Ave., L.A. 29, Calif., in the United States, and *World Forum*, *Health for All*, and many others overseas.

morning, take a warm bath first and follow it with the cold shower.

Exercises

Five or ten minutes—or even three—spent on a few well-selected exercises for keeping the spine "loose" and strengthening the abdominal muscles, after the morning bath and scrub, are a good investment for the day, especially for those who cannot spare time for a walk. Deep breathing (based on completely emptying the lungs rather than on straining to fill them) before an open window should be a regular part of the program for nonwalkers.

Remember that it will take a little time for the body to get accustomed to the change, so do not be discouraged if you have to wait for results. They are sure to come.

4 / *How to make the change*

Many people would like to test the Waerland diet on their own health but hesitate to take the step, fearing that the change from an ordinary "civilized" diet would be accompanied by unpleasant disturbances and that it is essential to attempt it only under expert guidance. Anyone who feels at all doubtful needs only to seek out some of the thousands who have carried out the transition by studying the Waerland literature and have attained health such as they never thought possible.

In this chapter I would like to discuss the problem of how to set about changing one's diet. The change-over must be carefully planned to suit each individual case, and consideration given to the kind of life and diet the patient has been used to and especially the state of the digestive organs. Those who have been living a healthy life already, to some extent, with a diet including a certain amount of raw food and wholemeal bread will usually find no difficulty in changing over to a lacto-vegetarian diet. A certain tiredness and lassitude may be felt during the first four to six weeks, because of the poisonous residues which have been latent in the tissues and are now thrown out into the bloodstream before being eliminated from the body. This is natural, but a reaction of this kind is not met in every case. If the person has not previously been constipated and has had plenty of fresh air and exercise, he will notice an immediate improvement in health and spirits.

Even those already in good health at the time of the change-over must, nevertheless, take care to drink plenty of liquids between meals. The quantities recommended are

1 pint first thing in the morning (preferably potato water or vegetable broth).

1 pint at midmorning and at midafternoon.

This plentiful intake of liquid and an insistence on three or four bowel movements daily are equally essential for the elimination of long-standing impurities from the body. If the bowel does not function unaided, it must be encouraged by the use of enemas, which are always beneficial during the period of readjustment to the new diet, making it easier and more effective. Double enemas every night for a couple of weeks may be safely taken, that is: first a small enema of about a pint of tepid water, followed immediately after ejection by a larger one of a quart.

It is important not to continue the large enemas too long, preferably not longer than about a month. After this a change can be made to small cool injections of about one pint. These may be continued as long as seems necessary, without doing any harm, as they have no relaxing effect. A small cool enema taken immediately after a meal (preferably the evening meal), when peristalsis is in full activity, is most efficacious. The cool (nearly cold) water causes a contraction of the rectal muscles which stimulates the large intestine into activity. If this is done every day at the same time, the bowel forms the habit of emptying itself at that time, and gradually less and less water will be required to induce the desired reaction until the enema is no longer required: the bowel has learned to act spontaneously.

Another important part of the change-over is the addition of linseed (flaxseed) and bran to the morning drink. Linseed contains a particularly beneficial oil which lubricates the mucous membrane of the intestines, and the bran carries the fluid into the great bowel (colon) and prevents the stools from becoming too hard. To enable the intestine to empty itself properly, the stools should be of the consistency of porridge.

We must take into account the fact that in practically everybody nowadays the bacterial flora of the colon has been so changed by years of living on devitalized foods that it is no longer able to break down the cellulose contained in raw vegetables. The first thing to be aimed at, therefore, is to cleanse the bowel thoroughly and then to introduce and cultivate the bacteria which are necessary for digesting and making use of the health-giving ingredients of a natural diet.

But how can we "cultivate" these useful bacteria?

It is quite simple. They are contained in sour milk. So we must eat plenty of sour milk and yogurt. We must start our day with sour milk and, in some form or other, it should accompany the vegetable meal. The same bacteria, so vital for our good health, are also found in sauerkraut. This is a popular dish in Germany and Switzerland and can be bought ready-prepared without salt in the health-food stores there. It is appetizing and delicious, adding piquancy to the meal, besides aiding digestion. It can be made at home in small quantities in this way:

> Finely shredded cabbage leaves; small quantity of juniper berries.
>
> Place the cabbage in layers in a wooden pail or earthenware crock, with a few juniper berries between the layers. Crush the cabbage by pounding it as each layer is added, until it is a compact mass. Place a weighted lid on the top and leave to stand. The juice of the cabbage should rise and cover the whole. After a day or two scum will have formed on the top and should be removed, the lid and weight washed each time. When no scum forms it will keep. It takes about a month before it is ready to eat. (Full recipe for large quantity on p. 206.)

If, during the change-over to the Waerland diet, people do not abide by the instructions already given to drink enough liquid and keep the bowels active, they often suffer from gases in the intestine, with griping pains and other discomforts. These unpleasant symptoms are due to the lack of proper bacteria and disappear as soon as these have been cultivated. A further aid to the process is to take milk sugar with the sour milk. The bacteria in affinity with raw vegetables thrive on the milk sugar and increase more rapidly.

But, most important of all, never again eat meat, fish, or eggs once you have decided on the new diet. Be consistent and keep to it a hundred per cent. It is futile to give with one hand and take back with the other, at the same time expecting to succeed. Each time you eat food encouraging to putrefactive bacteria, you let loose a war between the putrefactive ones and our friends the fermentative bacteria—and it takes several weeks to fight it to a conclusion.

A compromise between a faulty or deficient diet and one entirely composed of foods having positive nutritive value is, of course, better than a completely wrong diet. It is better to include in the ordinary civilized diet a certain amount of raw vegetables and fruit and wholemeal bread than to leave them out entirely. It is a step in the right direction, but it will not lead to anything like the high degree of health and vitality attained by so many out-and-outers through strict adherence to a health-building diet and harmonious way of life. It means, of course, avoiding everything that injures the body or disorganizes its functioning, including all stimulants and refined, devitalized foods.

Impaired digestive organs

The change-over is naturally more difficult for people whose organs have been impaired, as was the case with me. But precisely because I suffered from serious colitis for thirty-five years and had been unable all my life to digest proper, nourishing foods, and *in spite of this* was able to make the change, I am a living example of how it can be done, even with the most seriously damaged organs. Moreover, many of the patients I have since treated had such badly damaged organs that it did not seem possible that they could ever assimilate any nourishment, yet they, too, bear witness to the way in which impaired organs can be regenerated. We have even seen patients cured who had only a very small part of the stomach left after an operation. With great patience and perseverance the part that remained was enabled to function so efficiently that, mainly through raw diet, the patient eventually found his way back to health.

But each one of these patients had to find his own way, just as each one that we advise is treated individually. There are, however, certain basic lines to be followed when the change-over is complicated by imperfect or debilitated organs. I will briefly outline them here.

Fasting on raw juices

A fast with raw alkaline juices is the best way of assisting the change-over:

On waking: 1 pint of potato water or vegetable broth in which 2 tablespoons of agar-agar have been soaked overnight. All to be consumed.

Breakfast, Lunch & Dinner: A pint of liquid consisting of ⅔ juice of carrot (best) or other root vegetable, and ⅓ potato water or vegetable broth.

Midmorning & Afternoon: Two cups of herb tea.

Altogether about 2 to 2½ quarts of liquid is desirable for patients who have no heart or kidney trouble. Those who have must cut this down to 1½ quarts and drink very slowly. Enema morning and night.

Even a three-day fast makes the change easier. Five days is more useful and a week even better. Persons who have nervous trouble, overactive thyroid gland, tuberculosis, or heart disease, however, should not fast at all.

Those who have impaired digestive organs, who suffer from diarrhea, colitis, or other symptoms of reduced ability to assimilate food, should be extremely careful on changing over. In most cases there are sores on the mucous membrane to be healed, and debilitated, slackened intestines to be trained to work normally. These patients are encouraged to put on the armor of patience.

The first step, however, is always to give up meat, fish, and eggs and all denatured foods. In certain cases cooked vegetables must be permitted in conjunction with increasing quantities of raw juices or roots and green vegetables. The basis of nourishment should consist in the extremely easily digested potato, boiled without salt and, at first, peeled until the intestine is strong enough to deal with the skin, so rich in cellulose but so valuable. Sour milk in various forms should be introduced from the beginning even if the intestine reacts with diarrhea. For without sour milk we can never get a healthy bacterial flora in the bowel.

Spinach and carrots lose very little of their value when cooked, in contrast to all other roots and green vegetables, and are consequently invaluable to delicate digestions. Whole linseed, either raw in drinks or boiled for severe cases, is very healing for the mucous membrane of the intestines.

Impaired or diseased intestines cannot deal with wholemeal products. To begin with, rusks made from wheaten flour from which the bran has been extracted should be given and the patient slowly accustomed to wholemeal rusks and bread. Rusks are easier to digest than bread. Diarrhea is best checked by drinking a decoction of dried blueberries* or by a meal of rice boiled in water. The blueberries should be soaked overnight and boiled for twenty minutes in the morning. (Two heaping tablespoonfuls of blueberries to a quart of water.)

An excellent drink for delicate stomachs and intestines, which is both healing and nourishing, is our decoction of potatoes, linseed and bran.

Preparation: 1 lb. of potatoes cut in pieces and boiled in 3 pints of water for half an hour; 1¾ cups wheat bran and ⅜ cup linseed,† soaked overnight in 3 pints of hot water, then boiled for half an hour, the bran and linseed strained off and thrown away, the liquid being added to the potato water. Raw carrot juice should be added—from one tablespoonful to a small glass—as much as the patient is able to digest.

A cup of this decoction may be taken at each meal and also one or two cups as a drink between meals.

* Blueberries: in England called bilberries. The name, bilberries, is also used for some varieties of blueberries found from Maine, Michigan, and Oregon northward to Alaska and northeastern Canada. The Swedish variety is *Vaccinium myrtillus.*

† English equivalent is 6 tablespoons of wheat bran and 3 tablespoons of whole linseed.

Easy change-over diet for invalids

Morning drink: Decoction with carrot juice (as above) or, for diarrhea, with blueberry juice.

Midmorning & Afternoon: The same. Camomile tea as a change.

Breakfast: Sour milk (if possible, "long milk," * the most easily digested form of sour milk) with a small glass of carrot juice and crushed linseed.

Lunch: Potatoes, boiled in skins without salt, then peeled and eaten with a little butter, perhaps also a little whey cheese† and cottage cheese. "Long milk" (when available) or mild sour milk, rusks, and a little raw juice or decoction.

Dinner: Boiled vegetables, boiled potatoes or rice, a little milk and water if whole milk cannot be digested, rusks, butter.

Other variations: molino, or potato porridge. (See recipe, page 204.)

* See Glossary.

† The Swedish *mesost* and the Norwegian *gjetost* are made of whey from goat's milk. They are available in some parts of America, especially where there are many Scandinavians.

5 / *My own case history*

My start in life was handicapped by the fact that when I was born my mother was still suffering from the effects of puerperal fever after the birth of my sister the previous year. I was delicate from birth, a puny child with a low resistance to infection, easily tired, a poor sleeper, with little appetite and a weak digestion. I could not play and romp with the other children and was always conscious of my physical inferiority.

As a very young child I had several shocks which left their marks for years on my mind. One of these was a small operation for adenoids, insignificant in itself, but the surgeon had advised my parents not to prepare me at all for what was to happen. He arranged to take me by surprise in the nursery. It was too much for the nerves of a sensitive little child to find itself suddenly left alone at the mercy of two white-robed strangers and, without explanation or anesthetic, be seized and held while being forced to submit to an outrage. Terrible nightmares about white-clothed murderers pursued me afterwards for many years and there were many sleepless nights.

The next shock came shortly afterward, when I was five years old. I was sent away with a nurse to a mountain sanatorium in Norway. She did not understand how to calm a frightened little girl screaming in her sleep at night but punished me by slapping me and leaving me alone. The terror this treatment left in its wake was not easily erased from my childish mind.

Violent nosebleeds during the whole of my childhood and youth weakened me so much that I always had to carry twisted wads of cotton in my pocket. It usually meant going straight home to lie on my back with ice packs until the flow stopped. Not until, at eighteen, when both nostrils were cauterized, was I released from the constant dread of it. Naturally I was always anemic, pale, and pathetic. The various children's ailments attacked me more severely than they did my sisters and brothers, and during autumn, winter, and spring I was regularly haunted by catarrhal troubles, bronchitis, swollen tonsils, and disgusting colds and neuralgia.

When I was eleven I developed intestinal catarrh, which grew worse as time went on. We had a children's doctor who gave me his own pet remedy—bromide—which did no good. At fifteen I was allowed to accompany my parents on a visit to the Riviera, but I caught a cold on the way and spent the whole of our stay in a darkened hotel bedroom. My inflamed, mattery eyes could stand no light, my throat was sore, my head and ears ached. On our return after six weeks I was on the verge of a breakdown, and when the usual infections of the winter began I had a nervous collapse. I became extremely shy, wept day and night, and, if I had dared, would have taken my life. Several times I got up on the window sill at night to jump out, but at the last moment something always held me back. The will to live is the greatest help a sick person can have.

At this time I was sent to a sanatorium for six months. After that I had no further nervous trouble, but my other complaints persisted and grew even worse. Next to insomnia, my worst trouble was complete lack of appetite. I had a continuous nausea and had to force myself to swallow food. For days I had to lie in bed, unable to keep anything down. This meant severe malnutrition, and at thirteen my lungs became affected. I went about with a raised temperature which never was regularly normal—until, over thirty-three years later, I changed my diet.

All this time my sleeplessness continued. From fifteen years of age I was unable to sleep without opiates, which were, of course, continuous poison.

At seventeen I was acutely poisoned through eating some canned food and had to go to a hospital. I was treated by the famous Swedish stomach specialist Dr. Olin and spent five years in hospitals and sanatoria of his without avail. When I found that Dr. Olin was unable to help me, I turned to another well-known younger specialist, Dr. Nauckhoff, and for two years he treated me, most of the time in a hospital, but he could give me no help either. Both men were the King's physicians and of the highest repute.

After another four years I sought out a third famous Swedish specialist, Dr. Hedenius. He wanted to perform colostomy, immobilize the whole of the large intestine, and operatively insert an artificial outlet. Fortunately I refused to adopt his suggestion, which would have made me a complete invalid for life. Instead I went abroad to see if a change of climate would renew my strength. By the time I was twenty-four I weighed ninety-seven pounds and was six feet tall, had forty per cent hemoglobin, and was so weak that I often fainted. For many years I had from twenty to thirty painful bowel movements daily, passing blood and mucus all the time.

After several months in the South, I felt so much worse that I could no longer retain any food and decided to go home while I still had strength for the journey. I had now abandoned all hope of recovery.

On my way back through Berlin a friend persuaded me to go to a well-known physician, Professor Plesch, but he refused to have anything to do with me. He said I had come too late, that all my organs were impaired and I was starving to death. Not only my lungs and intestines, but my liver also had been ailing for ten years. With great trouble we were able to persuade this brilliant man, who had already achieved many miracles with hopeless cases, to take on mine also. For a whole year I was given his treatment, first at his own hospital in Berlin, then in Dresden, and finally for six months at a lung sanatorium in Davos.

It was essential to induce the digestive organs to resume their work. Therefore, to bring about a reaction and stimulate the metabolism and circulation, Professor Plesch prescribed very cold sitz (hip) baths. Every day I was placed for twenty long minutes in running water at a temperature of forty-six degress Fahrenheit and then massaged and packed around with hot-water bottles until the circulation and feeling were restored to the numbed tissues. Through this treatment the digestive system was so stimulated that I could again eat and retain a little food and thus gain strength. During this time I was being stuffed from morning till evening and doubled my weight in the course of a year.

After six months at Davos, my parents thought I had spent enough time in hospitals and sanatoria and took me home, in spite of protests from my doctors, who insisted that my lungs were not yet healed. I now married the friend who had introduced me to Professor Plesch and thereby restored me to life. Shortly afterward I was expecting a child. Then for four and a half months I suffered from continuous vomiting and lost forty-five pounds. At the confinement I had severe hemorrhages. Unfortunately we had hesitated for twelve hours before it was decided to operate. It was a case of placenta praevia,* and the baby and I both almost bled to death. At the women's hospital in Bern, I was operated on at the last moment by Professor Guggisberg, who performed a very complicated Caesarean. For many years afterward I suffered from catarrh of the bladder. As I was coming round after the anesthetic, an intolerable pain in my chest arose from a saline injection being given to replace the loss of blood.

My baby's head had been hurt during this difficult birth; it had been pinched and injured by the forceps. It was quite blue and had convulsions for several days. The professor gave us little hope and thought that neither of us would survive. "If the child does live," said he, "it will be

* Abnormal position of the placenta.

an idiot." Happily this prophecy proved incorrect. Although the doctors forbade me, I wanted to feed the child and insisted on trying to do so, but I had to give up when the glands in both breasts became infected and inflamed. I lay in a high fever, and a relapse of tuberculosis was diagnosed. This diagnosis was confirmed by Professor Sahli.

I was now sent up into the mountains for rest cures in various sanatoria and rented houses. Because I was so weak, the doctors forbade me to have another child. But I longed for more children, and when after four and a half years I was better, a second came. The confinement was long and difficult, followed again by a high fever. I began to feed the child, but after five days I had to stop because tuberculosis had again developed. The famous Professor Neumann of Vienna diagnosed it this time.

I was taken by ambulance to a health resort not far from Vienna, and arrived there with a septic phlebitis which forced me to lie motionless on my back for seven months. During this time I had three attacks of acute lung catarrh, once pleurisy, and once embolism. I cannot possibly describe how I suffered during those months. But at last the time came when I was able once more to sit for a minute on the edge of the bed and let my legs hang down. It was, however, months before I could drag myself across the room with the help of two canes. The way back to life after such a long and dangerous illness is often more distressing than the illness itself.

After this I was obliged to take frequent "cures," lying out of doors in the invigorating mountain air, and my health gradually improved. But after four or five years I had a serious attack of influenza with several relapses, and septic phlebitis followed again, this time in both legs. For six months I had to lie motionless on my back, suffering indescribably. My heart, which had hitherto been sound, was now so spent that I was obliged to take digitalis constantly.

But my love of life and the will to live saved me once more, bearing me along the uphill road back to life. I stayed in the mountains for several more years and finally returned to Sweden, still suffering from the same chronic complaints. Not unnaturally, the children also had low resistance and were a constant prey to diseases. None of us could stand town life, so we settled down in the country.

More than once my ovaries became inflamed, and repeated bleeding from the vagina forced me to undergo uncomfortable treatments. In 1938 I developed a form of angina. My tonsils had been removed when I was eighteen, giving poisons free play in my body, and I now got rheumatic fever. I was in bed for eight months, and during this time had five operations for abscesses in the jawbone. My long-standing migraine became acute, and I had blinding, nauseating attacks, intolerably painful, after which, even in the intervals, I was unable to read or write. This condition did not clear up entirely until a couple of years after I had begun the Waerland diet.

As I was not getting better from the rheumatic fever, I again went to the South, where a year in a warm climate helped me so far that I was able to return home to

Sweden. But my husband then fell a victim to an incurable sepsis and was seriously ill for half a year before he died. Soon after his death I had double pleurisy and was in bed for several months. When I was able to get up I felt wretched. During the many years of illness I had been through, an emphysematous condition of the lungs had established itself and was, according to medical science, incurable. The migraine was unbearable and I had a continuous headache even between attacks. The intestinal catarrh, insomnia, and all the other ailments cast a gloom over my whole life.

My daughter now contracted scarlet fever with dangerous complications and for three months hovered between life and death. The undue strain and anxiety told on me and brought on pneumonia, added to which the pus formations in my jawbone flared up again and a fresh series of operations became necessary. My heart had been enfeebled and degenerating for years; now I suffered from enlarged heart and weakness of the heart muscle.

It was while in this hopeless condition that I came across one of Are Waerland's books. When I had read to the end of it, it seemed as though scales had fallen from my eyes; a completely new conception of the problem of health and disease opened up. I decided to make a last desperate attempt to get well. I had nothing further to lose. But how was I to make the drastic change in diet? Never in my life had I been able to eat wholemeal bread, raw vegetables and raw fruit. It looked impossible, and yet I could see that here was my only road to salvation. So I persuaded myself to persevere with it.

In six months I had succeeded in healing the mucous membrane of the intestines and established a new and healthy bacterial flora in the colon by giving up all animal protein except milk, and gradually learned to digest a little sour milk. Step by step I struggled on in spite of difficult crises.

During this time I had to have three operations on my jaw in preparation for a big one: decay had set in and the whole of the right upper jawbone had to be scraped from ear to nose and a section of it removed. When the protracted and difficult operation was over, the surgeon, a well-known specialist in Stockholm, declared that as soon as I was strong enough it would have to be repeated as it had not been possible to remove the whole of the decayed part.

I had now progressed so far that I was cautiously trying to eat raw vegetables. This had a remarkable effect on me. My jaw healed up cleanly, the pus disappeared, and the second operation became unnecessary. Everything healed up splendidly. In two years I felt ten years younger. One after another, the various chronic diseases, declared incurable, were completely cured.

At last I had begun to live. About a year after the change of diet, however, I had the bad luck to fall off my bicycle. This resulted in a serious concussion of the brain and a fractured bone in one of my shoulders. I lay in bed for several weeks with a severe headache. But I got over this accident very quickly, indeed, in record time!

A year later I went to the Mediterranean and in a week had learned to swim. Before this I had not dreamed that I should ever be able to swim. But I presumed too far. It was late autumn and we had a ten-minutes' walk in wet bathing clothes. In my new enthusiasm I strained my weak heart and caught double pneumonia. But what a difference! This time I recovered in three weeks. Whereas, formerly the slightest cold had meant long-drawn-out complications and weakness, I now had the resilience of a steel spring. Only my heart would not quiet down.

A great task lay before me. My one great desire was to translate Are Waerland's most important book, *In the Cauldron of Disease*, from English into German. I worked from very early in the morning to late at night. When the translation was finished I had a breakdown and was taken by ambulance to Switzerland. I went to a sanatorium where I could have the Waerland diet. There it was found that I had bad ruptures in the heart muscle. Yet, after only a month's rest on the diet I recovered and was able to take up my work again.

Two years later I caught a germ from a patient who was suffering from a new virus disease known as "Italian sickness." It was a serious type of pneumonia, with the same choking symptoms as in whooping cough, so that the patient almost suffocated. Because it was such a new virus, the body had no antitoxins to combat it, and all the new wonder drugs such as penicillin and aureomycin had no effect. I lay at home in a high fever for two weeks. As my temperature rose above 104°, Dr. Gentz, the best lung specialist in Stockholm, ordered me to be taken at once to a hospital and given oxygen. There was hardly a spot in my lungs which was not affected. "Now, Mrs. Waerland," said the doctor, "you must show what your diet is worth," and he let me decide for myself how I should be treated. I gave myself a semi-fast, taking only yogurt and raw juices. The result was that I went home five weeks later *healed and without fever,* although a little weak. After a further month, I went to the doctor's consulting room. He described my cure as a miracle and gave our diet full credit for it.

In the autumn of 1950 I took on the direction of our Health Center at Kiholm. I had an enormous burden of work, including heavy physical tasks, with the result that during that winter I lost thirty-three pounds. It was a wonder that my back could stand all this strain. Ever since childhood I had suffered from backache owing to weakness of the spine aggravated by so much lying in bed. This had caused a deformity. All the osteopaths I had consulted had declared the condition incurable. I still have two infirmities: a deformed spine and dropped digestive organs.

In the middle of April, 1951, I started straight from my work at Kiholm on a six weeks' lecture tour of Switzerland and Germany. The hotels were unheated and the overcrowded lecture halls so hot that I was continually being soaked with perspiration. Added to this was the great strain of the constant traveling and the late evenings. A cold was inevitable, but I had to keep my engagements and could not take any rest. When the tour was over I broke down with catarrh of both lungs and irritation of the pleura. I had to stay in bed for a month in Hamburg.

But again I made a remarkably quick recovery, and two

weeks later I was in the midst of work directing with Are Waerland the international courses at Kiholm.

During all the years I have lived on the Waerland diet I have been able to do the work of a whole lifetime, thanks to the renewed health, energy, and joy which have come to me through this way of life.

6 / *The physiologically correct fast*

A properly carried-out fast must never be confused with "starving." It is always the shortest cut to health and is our most effective weapon in the fight against disease. Relieved of the work of digestion, the body is able to concentrate all its energies on dissolving and eliminating the stagnant residues from the tissues. This is the point where the internal "spring house cleaning" begins, which is the first essential step on the way back to health.

During the fast the cleansing process must be assisted in every way by enemas or colonic irrigation; also, whereever possible, by some form of *Sauna,** or steam bath, and exercise in the fresh air.

At all the sanatoria run on the Waerland lines in Sweden, Germany, and Switzerland, a fast is the most important factor in the treatment. It is amazing how quickly the body can rid itself of accumulated toxins when unencumbered by the work of digestion. A fast on raw juices is usually carried out without any unpleasant sensations, although the patient may feel slightly hungry during the first three days. In isolated cases, where the organism has become overloaded with toxins, there may even be some nausea, but this soon passes. After these initial disturb-

* See Glossary.

ances the fasting goes on with increasingly pleasant sensations of ease and well-being. The symptoms of disease disappear more and more as the blood and tissues are cleansed. A fast like this can be likened to a rebirth.

If the patient does not take a sufficient quantity of fluids, the poisons which have been gathering up in the tissues will overflow into the bloodstream. They cannot be carried away in the natural way by the organs of elimination, *which are unable to function without fluids.* The poisons will then be forced to find a way out through the skin in the form of eruptions, boils, and sores. The fast, which should be pleasant, will become a nightmare, more painful than the disease, and will do very little to bring the sufferer nearer his goal.

Most of the experts on fasting understand the need for fluids but, unfortunately, very few know the best way of carrying out a fast in a physiologically co-operative manner. Many of them still allow their patients to fast on water only, or on fruit juices and teas. It is true that some good is done by cutting out the work of the digestion, but experience and science have now taught us that even better results can be achieved.

Dr. Ragnar Berg, the well-known nutritionist, has carried out extensive tests in connection with fasting and has established the fact that, during a fast on fruit juice or water, the excessive acidity of the body is increased so much that it loses its ability to dissolve the accumulated toxins. The urine becomes dark and thick, a condition which is interpreted by an inexperienced person as an indication of copious excretion of poisons. This is a mistake.

On the contrary, the clear, pale urine of a person fasting on raw alkaline vegetable juices contains a far larger proportion of residues which have been set free by the solvent and neutralizing properties of the fluids taken.

In order to gain the greatest possible benefit from a fast, the body must have a plentiful supply of raw alkaline juices.

When I took over the direction of the Kiholm Health Center in the autumn of 1950, I immediately introduced fasting on alkaline raw juices without having heard of Dr. Berg's researches. In doing so, I was led, as in several other cases, by a certain instinct which was proved correct by my own practical results and later confirmed by Dr. Ragnar Berg's findings. All these fasts were successful.

Since that time I have watched over hundreds of fasting patients, many of whom had already tried a water or fruit-juice fast. They all declared that my fast had been a revelation. They had never imagined that a fast could be accompanied by such a feeling of physical ease and well-being and alertness of brain.

With regard to the treatment of cancer by fasting, there is some diversity of opinion among the specialists in natural healing. Great authorities such as Dr. Johannes Kuhl in Germany and Dr. Gerson in America prescribe fasting on raw alkaline juices, and my own experience has been that precisely in such cases a fast is often the only effective remedy. Even in so-called "hopeless" cases, wonderful results have been achieved by a physiologically planned fast which uses the body's own resources in dealing with the diseased tissues.

In advanced cases of cancer, where there is no possible hope of recovery, a fast on these lines, if begun in time, will do much to help the patient toward an easier, less painful death.

In practically every disease the highway to health is fasting plus other forms of encouragement given for the elimination of poisons. But, in cases where the heart or kidneys are defective, or there is nervousness, neurasthenia, goiter, or tuberculosis, fasting may have to be avoided.

I am looking forward to the day when these methods may be scientifically tested and their value proved in some of the larger hospitals.

7 / *Rheumatism, gout, and arthritis*

In describing the way back to health from various forms of disease, it seems natural to begin with the rheumatic diseases, about which Are Waerland wrote and lectured so much. These are the commonest of all complaints, and we have found that they respond very readily to our treatment. Among the cases cured through a change of diet, we have records of many patients who were crippled by arthritis, helpless, and confined to a wheel chair. That cases of such severity can be helped, the pain relieved, and the distorted limbs restored to more natural forms is one of the miracles of nature.

At the beginning of Waerland's activity in Sweden, in the year 1937, when he traveled all over the country giving his first rousing lectures, and wrote his first revolutionary articles, many wretched rheumatic sufferers made a bold bid to break with old habits and prejudices and were rewarded by regaining their health. At that time little had been done in the sphere of dietetic therapy, and the ordinary Waerland diet* (for those in good health) was used for all diseases, generally with excellent results. It was not until ten years later that the original diet began to be adapted for specialized treatment of specific dis-

* See Chapter 3.

eases, thereby achieving much quicker and better results. Without these specific modifications the Waerland system would not have been accepted by the biologists of the German medical profession as it is today.

How are these results obtained?

Overacidity is one of the symptoms found in all rheumatic subjects without exception. This condition is the first thing to correct, and that is why the diet must be highly alkaline, including two rawkost* meals daily, while avoiding all acid-forming foods, especially cereals and fruits.

We have found repeatedly, in all localities, that fresh fruits and cereals have a retarding effect in the treatment of rheumatic complaints. This has been confirmed over and over again when a patient, having got well established on the road to recovery, has had a relapse and a return to his aches and pains after eating fresh, raw fruit. Our advice, therefore, to all rheumatic subjects is "Beware of fruit until all the symptoms have departed." Even for some time afterward it is necessary to be careful. The same advice applies to bread, kruska, and sprouted wheat grains.

In treating acute cases, when the body is defending it-

* Rawkost: Literally, raw food. The rawkost meal consists of a large raw-vegetable salad including both root and green leaf vegetables, up to a pound of potatoes cooked in their skins and the skins eaten, and sour milk. You may also eat a slice of whole-grain bread, but do not overdo the bread, because this is intended to be the main alkaline meal of the day. You may eat a piece of raw potato also, if you wish. Do not add fruits to this vegetable meal.

self by fever, we avoid all physical treatment in the form of baths, etc., and give the patient complete rest, while he is fasting in bed. The same precautions must be taken where the heart is affected. If the heart has been strained, it must be spared in every possible way, and can also be strengthened by taking tincture of Crataegus. Many patients have toned up the action of the heart by taking this harmless homeopathic remedy from nature's rich store. At this acute stage, perspiration plays an important part in the elimination of acids and other toxins. The skin should be assisted by washing the body with a cloth dipped in luke warm water. This washing may be done standing by a wash basin or in bed. It removes the acrid body odor which is typical of rheumatic conditions. Careful and wise assistance given to all the recuperative forces of the body never fails to bring better results.

Cold showers are not brought into use until the patient has almost recovered.

In chronic cases warm soda baths (see p. 202) followed by perspiring in bed are a very useful form of treatment. The purpose of the baths is to promote perspiration, but here again, great caution must be oberved if the patient has a weak heart. After perspiring, the patient should be sponged with tepid water and then lie in bed for at least two hours. It is best not to leave the patient alone while perspiring and the pulse should be checked from time to time.

The case of Dr. Rudolf Jansa

Dr. Jansa is a well-known dental surgeon in Bremen, employing seven assistants in his clinic. He is a man of about fifty, now full of vitality.

His rheumatic troubles began twenty years ago with painful swelling of the feet, particularly in the big toes. No one at that time recognized the signs of incipient gout. Both Dr. Jansa himself and the doctors he consulted blamed his profession, and fourteen different kinds of apparatus for the feet were tried for years, even to the extent of a support for the hips, but without the slightest results. The pain and swelling only became worse. Dr. Jansa tried all the methods of treatment offered by the various reform movements then known in Germany. He tried different types of fasting and vegetarian food reform, but all in vain.

As his condition grew worse, an examination of the blood showed unusually high uric acid content. Dr. Jansa was now being treated by a well-known homeopath, Dr. Schültz, and went into his hospital several times during bouts of unusual severity, but no improvement was made. In 1939 a fast of twenty-one days under the supervision of Rudolf Just, the specialist in fasting, made no permanent improvement, and every year his condition became worse. During the war he was, of course, exempted from military service and tried to carry on his profession, but it became increasingly difficult for him to keep going. He says that no one who has not gone through it can possibly imagine what a martyrdom he had to endure. Again, from 1944 to 1948 he went to all the best authorities in Germany and tried their methods, following their advice and instructions in every detail, including all kinds of injections and drugs, even snake venom.

Finally he was obliged to have a special chair made, as he was unable to stand and had to do his work sitting down. For years he was unable to bear shoes on his feet, and the pain was so bad that he sought refuge in drugs.

This final phase of the disease was indescribably agonizing. The greatest authorities of the medical profession declared that his case was completely hopeless. Professor Sudeks, of Hamburg, summarized his opinion in these words: "I cannot help you. What you are suffering from is typical gout in such an acute form that I have seldom seen anything like it."

But Dr. Jansa did not entirely abandon hope and tried desperately to find a straw to cling to. Just then, when there was apparently no hope, Are Waerland came from Sweden to lecture in Bremen. Dr. Jansa had heard something of the results of the Waerland diet and decided to make a final effort to see if a change of diet would overcome his terrible disease. With unspeakable difficulty he got himself taken to the lecture. Afterward, with iron persistency and consistency, he carried out the new diet. Month after month he struggled on, step by step. He knew that it would take patience and perseverance and did not lose courage when the attacks came. His friends and patients followed the experiment with keen interest and at last, after months of adjustment and readjustment, the pain began to lessen and the attacks came at longer intervals. Finally they ceased altogether.

Dr. Jansa has changed over to the Waerland diet. Four years after the change, he had undergone a complete transformation and been restored to life with all its possibilities. He now is able to stand for ten hours every day, and the special chair he had made has become superfluous. He is playing tennis again with all his old agility and suppleness, and he says he has never felt so well and full of vitality as now. He goes in for all kinds of outdoor pursuits, including long camping trips in southern Europe.

Our first bed patient at Kiholm came to us at the end of August, 1950. He arrived in an ambulance unheralded while the house was being cleaned after the summer courses and made ready for the winter months. The man, Birger Ohman, aged 38, was lifted out on a stretcher. He was thin as a skeleton, and his face and body were covered with boils and sores. He had heard of Kiholm and the wonderful results achieved with the Waerland diet, and now in despair he grasped at what seemed to be the last straw, the last possible hope of relief. Probably uncertain that we would receive anyone so seriously ill, he had not notified us beforehand.

At first it did seem impossible to receive him, but we soon realized that he would be lost if we did not take charge of him, so it was decided to take him in and try, by every possible means, to save his life.

Members of the staff were taken from other work and

sat at his bedside day and night, feeding him by teaspoonfuls on raw vegetable juices, mostly carrot, while enemas were used to promote elimination via the bowels.

The patient was in constant pain and hardly slept at all. His heart was badly affected and he had difficulty in breathing, owing to inflamed lungs and pleurisy. During the past five years he had spent long periods in hospitals, his history of suffering having begun with arthritis, for which all the regular treatments were tried, including gold injections. Finally two transplantations of pituitary gland were undertaken, whereupon he developed sores and boils all over his body. The diagnosis now read: "Severe arthritis, severe heart trouble, and incurable psoriasis."

It was in this state that he came to us. Our problem was how to rid this highly toxic organism of its poisons without straining the gravely affected heart.

The regenerating forces of nature are, however, astonishing if only they are given sufficient backing. In two or three weeks the pain had gone, except in the feet, and sleep and appetite were returning, the latter gradually becoming ravenous hunger. The eruptions gradually cleared up, and after a few months the patient had a beautiful new skin. In two months from the time he arrived, he was able to get up, and by the end of November he was taking walks on the ice with the support of a chair sled (*sparkstötting*).

At Christmas he went home, where he was received as one risen from the dead. Nobody could understand how the miracle had come about.

In January he returned to Kiholm for a further few months' treatment and in the autumn came back again, but this time to work for us. He was then in perfect health, his terrible illness only an evil memory. Eager to make up for all that he had missed, he bought a motorcycle, which he rode on icy, snow-covered roads, and it was not long before he had an accident one dark night, when he crashed and broke his hip. He was operated on in a hospital, but his newly gained health stood him in good stead and he was soon on his feet again and able to return to work.

Ture E., a man of 35, was another so-called hopeless case. He was suffering from arthritis and severe edema. His eyes were mere slits in a face so swollen as to be unrecognizable, and his legs swelled, as he tried to use them, into shapeless stumps. He, too, had wandered from hospital to hospital, having undergone all the various treatments of orthodox medicine, including injections of arsenic and sulphur. Finally his kidneys had been ruined by gold injections, and severe Bright's disease had developed. His last examination had registered ten promilles (albumin). Both knees had been operated on for discharges, besides which he had had double pneumonia with pleurisy. The diagnosis was "Chronic, incurable Bright's disease, severe heart trouble and severe arthritis."

It is only in extreme cases that I allow patients with heart trouble to fast. Usually in such cases they are put on the limited diet (see p. 201), a kind of semi-fast which has a very good cleansing effect. But some cases are so bad that one has to take the risk of a complete fast with raw alkaline juices. This was one.

Ture E. still possessed great recuperative powers. In ten days the edema had disappeared. Naturally he was not allowed to drink as much as ordinary fasting patients but was restricted to two and a half pints daily, the amount usually found suitable for patients with weak hearts or reduced kidney function. But even these patients must gradually train themselves to increase the amount, since only a liberal intake of fluids will keep the organs of elimination functioning properly.

Ture E. began to go up and down stairs without his legs becoming swollen, and his face returned to normal proportions. After thirteen days' fasting an examination showed a reduction of albumin to 1.4 promilles (albumin) and, after another week, 0.3 promilles. Radiant with joy and hardly able to realize his "miracle," he went home.

Among Waerlandists in various parts of the world—not only in the North—innumerable cases will be found of rheumatic sufferers who have found their way back to health by a change of diet in the same way as the three I have described.

Treatment for rheumatic diseases and arthritis

The same two basic causes give rise to the diseases in this group as to most others: (1) The poisoning of the whole organism by stagnating residues; (2) The deficiency of important elements of nutrition. In the first instance the poisoning is caused by our unnatural food and unhealthful way of living, with resultant constipation. The fundamental causes of constipation are, in fact, faulty diet, insufficient fluids, too little exercise, and lack of internal hygiene. In the second instance we have only to compare our modern diet with that of our biological forefathers (who, according to Sir Arthur Keith, lived 25 million years in the trees on a diet of leaves, grains, fruits, grasses, and nuts which, by its very nature, was the means of determining and building up the human digestive organs) to see that our modern civilized diet is lacking in many of the essentials demanded by the human body, such as minerals, fats, carbohydrates, proteins, and vitamins—*in organic, living form.*

Sufficient salt in the form of sodium chloride is contained in this natural food to make the addition of commercial salt unnecessary and harmful. This silts up in the tissues, causing them to retain large quantities of liquid. Salt must therefore disappear from our kitchens. Practical experiments have indicated that ordinary salt is one of the chief causes of rheumatic complaints.

Rheumatic patients all suffer from overacidity. They should, therefore, live on a highly alkaline diet. (See p. 202.) In the first stage of acute rheumatism, or if there is fever, no physical treatment should be given, but when the acute stage is over, warm soda baths (2 lbs. of washing soda to a bath), followed by perspiration in bed, are very beneficial. Commencing at a temperature of 99° F., the patient lies in the bath for 15 minutes, during which hot water is added until the temperature has reached 104° F., if the patient's heart can stand it. Perspiration should begin while in the bath and then continue in bed for about half an hour. Each case must, of course, be judged individually.

Both during the fast, which is invaluable in these diseases, and afterward, it is highly important that the patient's bowels should be kept active. During the fast an enema should be given night and morning. Rheumatic patients always fast on alkaline juices. (See instructions for fasting, and for breaking the fast, on p. 200.) As always, in cases where the heart or kidneys, or both, are defective, or there is nervousness, neurasthenia, goiter, or tuberculosis, fasting may have to be avoided.

Diet sheet for rheumatic patients

On Waking: Vegetable decoction with bran and linseed (see p. 199), "Excelsior."

Breakfast: Some form of sour milk with potato porridge. Instead of fruit: raw juice from root or green vegetables. For a change: figs. Suitable adjuncts: milk sugar and if desired, dried powdered nettles or rose hips, strewn on top of the sour milk (see recipe p. 207).

Midmorning and Afternoon: Herb tea, preferably from horsetail (*Equisetum arvense*).

Lunch: Raw vegetables of all kinds *except onions, horseradish, paprika, and everything strong and sharp, and leeks.* Plenty of potatoes cooked in jackets and a raw potato. Sour milk (long milk is best), unsalted butter, raw juices—mainly from carrot and celery or celeriac. No ordinary bread at first, only the special bread for rheumatics (recipe p. 195), and no cheese except whey and cottage cheese.

Supper: The same menu as at midday or, for a change, potato porridge or molino (recipe p. 204), applesauce or other stewed fruit, and sweet milk; butter, whey or cottage cheese, rheumatic bread. No ordinary bread or kruska.

To be avoided: All fruit except sweet, dried fruit. (Later, when the patient is better, sweet fresh fruit will be allowed.) Cereals and strongly flavored roots, such as onion, garlic, horse-radish. (In some cases exception is made for garlic.)

8 / *Asthma*

Diseases can be classified under two main groups, functional and organic. Asthma is a functional disease. Usually no organic fault is found in asthmatics which could produce such uncomfortable symptoms. It is typified by periodic attacks of breathlessness caused by contraction of the muscles of the fine air passages. These attacks usually occur at night. The shortness of breath becomes so acute that the patient has to sit up to overcome the feeling of suffocation. Fresh, pure air is the first essential when this happens.

The periodic return of these suffocating attacks indicates an accumulation of poisons in the body. When the organs of elimination are unable to do their work of carrying off residues quickly enough, these stagnate in the body and culminate in an attack.

Combustion—burning up—is the fundamental life process. Just as the fire burning on our hearth produces smoke and ashes—the "products of combustion"—so the body has its own "ashes and smoke" in the form of gases, which are eliminated through the lungs and skin, and less volatile substances which are carried off by the bowels and kidneys. The smaller the amount of worthless substances we introduce into the body and the sooner the products of combustion pass out of it, the better all our organs are able to function and the healthier we are. Health depends on all the life forces of the body being able to go on as nature intended; otherwise toxins and "ashes" will pile up in the organs and tissues, giving rise to the many and varied symptoms of disease. It is the derangement of the functioning of our organs which causes all these diseases.

Asthma and the whole group of respiratory diseases, including bronchitis and colds, are typical examples of this. So many poisonous residues are allowed to gather and stagnate in the bodies of people who have become over "civilized" to the extent of eating unsuitable food and in other ways habitually ignoring the laws of nature, that it only requires a sudden severe chilling of the skin to call forth colds or other disease symptoms.

Evidences of this are everywhere. Colds and all the diseases of this group amount to a desperate effort on the part of the body to rid itself of accumulated toxins. Anyone can prove this by his own experience if he consistently re-plans his diet and habits of life, avoiding as far as possible everything which will tend to hold up residues in the body and disorganize its functioning. Colds and allied complaints are the first to disappear when the change of diet has been made, and subsequently the other functional disturbances go, too.

From this it is clear that an asthmatic subject, especially, must live in fresh air and avoid all unnatural foods and luxuries. For in this case the toxicity of the body is already so high that the organism cannot cope with any more. Through chronic overstrain the internal functioning of the glands has been seriously deranged.

The most effective way to restore normal functioning and rid the body of toxins is by fasting. But, because asthma is an obstinate complaint, it may take several rather long fasts which must be carried out with alkaline juices, vegetable broth and special herb teas. (See instructions for fasting, p. 200.)

Diet for asthmatics

This is similar to the diet for rheumatic subjects. The asthmatic, however, usually can take fruit and should have as much onion and garlic as he can manage. He should avoid sweet milk and milk products which tend to encourage the formation of mucus. On the other hand, sour milk and homemade curd cheese are allowable. The daily plan of meals should be the following:

On waking: Morning drink (see various recipes).

Breakfast: Sour milk; fresh fruit and, if desired, a little dried fruit as well—currants, raisins, etc.—and the usual adjuncts to the sour milk.

Midmorning and Afternoon: Herb tea.

Lunch and Supper: Rawkost meal: raw grated roots and salads; sour milk; very little wholemeal bread. Butter should be replaced by cold-pressed oils,* regular cheese by cottage (curd) cheese, and bread reduced to one slice of whole grain bread per day. The spe-

* See Glossary.

cial bread for rheumatics is permitted. The most suitable teas are horsetail, coltsfoot, and camomile.

Asthmatic subjects are very sensitive to all kinds of dampness, whether of clothing or in the air. They feel best and recover most quickly in a mountain climate where the air is light and dry.

Proper functioning of the bowels is of supreme importance in this toxic condition. The asthmatic patient must therefore take care that the bowels move three times daily. Failing this a cool, one-pint enema after the main meals must be resorted to.

Cold sponge baths followed by thorough dry brushing all over the body are necessary to promote activity of the skin. The patient needs as much exercise as possible in the fresh air and should always sleep with open windows. Deep breathing exercises will help, but the patient must learn to breathe in the proper, physiological way, without straining or forcing.

At Kiholm (Sweden) and at other sanatoria where I worked abroad, we have had very good results with asthma patients. In all cases it was the fasting which did the most good, even where the patient was emaciated and one would not have expected him to be able to stand up to such a drastic treatment.

There are two types of asthmatic subject, the fat, puffy type and the thin, emaciated one. It is often easier to get results with the fat type, as the reduction in weight during a fast is an enormous relief and with each period of fasting the patient grows lighter and more active.

Among the many cases of asthma we have encountered,

two are outstanding. These patients found their own way back to health with only the advice of a friend or some Waerland literature to guide them.

Lennart Hallberg had been a streetcar conductor in Gothenburg for a year when, at the age of thirty, his tale of suffering began. As in so many other cases, it started with constipation. He went to doctors, was given medicine and diet sheets, but none of the doctors forbade him to smoke. The misuse of nicotine lowered his resistance and, owing to constipation, the toxins in the body accumulated. A succession of colds was followed by severe and prolonged bouts of bronchial catarrh which wore away his strength. The doctors prescribed more and stronger drugs—and then the asthma began. The attacks became more frequent and severe and finally Hallberg was unfit for work. The doctors were obliged to resort to injections, but the effect of these soon wore off. The patient had to visit the hospital two or three times a week. For eight months of the year he was unable to work, and the anxiety and worry about money began to affect his nerves. His wife had been earning their keep and looking after him, often being up all night during his suffocating attacks, but finally she broke down and had to go away for treatment herself.

Left alone, despairing, and ill, Hallberg wandered about the streets at night. He could not lie in bed because of the attacks. Sometimes he went down to the harbor and was tempted to seek liberation by a plunge into the dark water.

In this desperate condition he happened to meet one of

his mates who was a Waerlandist. This friend persuaded him to try a change of diet, and although he was afraid he would not be able to stand the strange foods, he soon found that his fears were groundless and the diet suited him excellently. He began to study the Waerland literature, and then Are Waerland came to Gothenburg to lecture. This meeting turned the scale. The will to live was aroused in the sick man and he saw clearly the path that would lead him to health. He understood, however, that he would have to go through several acute crises and that only by slow degrees, in stages, could his health be built up. He had three serious relapses, the last one being the worst. The doctor who had to be called in found his heart so weak that he was prepared for the end. Nevertheless, Life won the battle and the great work of regeneration began.

Hallberg now lived on a highly alkaline diet and had an enema night and morning. Slowly the attacks grew less severe, with longer intervals between. At last he was able to go to work again and after that he had no further relapses. He was even able to work overtime without getting exhausted, and this man, who had scarcely been able to drag himself along, soon found himself running three to four kilometers (2-2½ miles) without effort.

He had learned something that is infinitely important for all of us: to know his own body and the laws which govern its health—and he had become his own physician.

Wilhelm Friberg, the second outstanding case, had a similar experience of which he wrote recently to me from Finland.

His father had died of asthma and during the last year of his life had such difficulty in breathing that he could not lie down at all but had to spend his nights in a rocking chair. Wilhelm's brother, too, had died, aged 30, of asthma aggravated by an attack of pneumonia.

Friberg was 39 when, in 1928, his asthma developed. For twenty years he consulted doctor after doctor but none of them could help him, each year the verdict being more gloomy, and finally he was told there was no prospect whatever of recovery.

In 1948 he read an account in a Finnish newspaper of one of Are Waerland's lectures. He was skeptical but decided to try a change of diet. He had nothing to lose since he, too, had reached the stage of sitting up all night, but he was still able to drag himself to work by day. He was a rent collector and only the hours spent out of doors had saved him from having to give in long before.

At first, on changing over to the Waerland diet, he had the usual reaction in which the alkaline foods dissolved and precipitated the toxic residues in the tissues. These were carried in the bloodstream to the eliminative organs, which lost no time in expelling them from the body. One of the "exits" sought by impurities was through the skin, by means of a weeping rash on his face. Unfortunately, Friberg did not know about fasting. If he had taken that short cut he might have saved himself two painful years. It was three years before he was quite well, but since then there has been no relapse. He is now sixty-five and in perfect health.

These two "hopeless" cases clearly show that the life

forces within us are infinitely strong and, if only we give them free play, can work miracles. But only on condition that we co-operate with the regenerative forces and do not hamper them.

9 / Cancer

The greatest problem of our time is the ever-widening incidence of cancer, a disease of civilization, unknown among healthy, primitive races. Every sixth person dies from some form of this painful disease. Orthodox medicine has so far made little headway in mastering its ravages. Surgery often has disastrous consequences in malignant cases, when the removal of one growth releases the poisons into the bloodstream and, after a time, fresh tumors appear in other parts of the body. Similarly, X-ray and radium treatments often damage the still-healthy surrounding cells.

In spite of the profound researches and untiring endeavor of academic medicine, the statistics given at a recent conference on cancer showed the following results of operations and radiation treatment:

82% of all cancer cases treated die within 6 months to 5 years;
16% die later but also of cancer;
2% are cured by radiation-surgery.

Recent American statistics showed that the following percentages of all cancer cases were not curable by orthodox methods:

96% cancer of stomach and intestines;
65% cancer of the breast;

86% cancer of the bowel;
85% cancer of the uterus.

This means that these high percentages of cancer sufferers die within five years of the time that treatment has begun.

The great German authority in the field of cancer research, Professor Bauer of Heidelberg, clearly recognizes that an entirely new approach will have to be made. Many other authorities, such as Dr. Johannes Kuhl, have come to the same conclusion. Both Dr. Kuhl and Professor H. Kurten of Munich point to the part played by lactic acid in the cause and cure of cancer. In his very interesting writings* Dr. Kuhl openly disapproves of the use of X-ray and hormone treatment, and also of synthetic vitamins.

Orthodox medicine has hitherto paid insufficient attention to the usually long preliminary stage of the disease before the tumor develops, the period when the body is slowly being poisoned by wrong foods and harmful luxuries. Dr. Kuhl, on the other hand, and many modern biologists working on cancer research have come to the same view as Are Waerland, namely, that *the growth is the end product of a long pathological process of development.*

Dr. Kuhl and Are Waerland are both equally convinced that cancer diseases originate through poisoning of the cells. Kuhl's theory is that, when the metabolism is upset, a pathological quantity of lactic acid is developed. In its

* *Schach dem Krebs,* Johannes Kuhl, M.D., Ph.D., Humata Verlag, 1954, Berne, Switzerland. Also: *Arzneind Ernährungs Behandlung gutartiger und bösartiger Geschwülste.*

fight against the toxins of faulty metabolism the body summons all its strength for the regeneration of the damaged cells, and for this purpose it produces lactic acid. As the increasing poisoning impedes the regenerative process, the body continues to produce lactic acid in more and more pathological quantities. In this way the cells are prevented from developing and reaching maturity and, although continuing to increase, they degenerate into a morbid and exaggerated growth. The tumor is the end product of this struggle, the result of an accretion of immature cells arrested in oxidation. This frantic endeavor to rebuild with new cells shows the indomitable will-to-live of the human organism before it is finally overcome by disease.

Are Waerland describes this warfare in similar terms. He, also, refers to the uninhibited, unnatural growth of the poisoned cells and calls them "marauders running riot in the cell kingdom."

In his treatment of cancer, Dr. Kuhl adheres to the isopathic principle which is the fundamental principle of homeopathy, namely, that "the devil must be driven out by Beelzebub." He therefore gives his patients lactic acid in order to produce a particular reaction and so help the body to rid itself of the superfluous and harmful quantities of this substance. Simultaneously he introduces foods containing natural, organic minerals and vitamins, vital to the cells and the process of fermentation. In common with Dr. Gerson of New York, one of the best-known authorities in the field of nutrition, he also advocates fasting on raw alkaline juices supplemented by extra vitamin B.

The therapeutic methods of both Dr. Kuhl and Dr. Gerson coincide in the main with ours, and may be taken as a valuable corroboration of the Waerland principles. The new biological view of the causes and treatment of disease is being adopted more and more by modern research workers in the field of nutrition. The deeper understanding of the laws of nature which we are seeking to interpret is steadily growing in the world of medicine and will eventually revolutionize the whole conception of disease and its treatment.

Modern medical science now recognizes the catastrophic consequences of the adulteration and devitalization of commercialized foodstuffs, and is beginning to see the connection between the increase in cancer incidence and the preserving, refining, and coloring of our foods.

Because carbohydrates are the raw materials of lactic acid, Dr. Kuhl recommends, as the first prophylactic measure against the formation of pathological quantities of lactic acid, a radical cutting down (or even complete avoidance) of all foods which contain carbohydrates in denatured form—chiefly white sugar and refined flour. He also establishes the fact that, when we live on denatured foods which have, of course, lost their own organic ferments our body reacts with an increase of white blood corpuscles. This is a purely protective measure which has been confirmed by many scientists. Does not this reaction clearly show what an important part the quality of our food plays in the working of our bodies and our health, and in the fundamental cause of the diseases of civilization?

Dr. Kuhl obtained excellent results with a diet of raw vegetables and lactic-acid products in the treatment of cancerous diseases. In the same way, so-called "hopeless" cases have been cured by Waerland methods. What seems to be an unfathomable miracle is, in fact, only the result of understanding nature and obeying her laws.

I will now describe some cases of cancer which have completely recovered by means of the Waerland therapy.

Frau M. Lingenfelder, of Munich, the wife of a well-known physician and, herself, a domestic-science teacher experienced in dietetics, had for many years been following a recognized system of reformed diet. She had always had an open mind for new discoveries and research in the realm of nature cure and had, to the best of her ability, obeyed the laws of health. In spite of her scientific training in the processes of nutrition, however, she was always constipated and always tired and had unbearable headaches.

In 1948 a tumor in the uterus was diagnosed and X-ray castration was resorted to. She underwent twenty painful radiations which increasingly caused burns on the skin. After this a radium insertion in the uterus was given under narcosis. She had to lie motionless for fifty hours with the radium plate in the uterus, enduring terrible pain from the burn blisters, which afterward turned to suppurating sores. Her bladder ceased to function and a catheter had to be used. For many weeks she lay in bed tortured and exhausted. She could not digest any food, the sores would not heal, and it was months before she was able to think of getting up.

In October, 1949, she had an inflamed condition of the throat and took one of the sulphonamide drugs. This was followed by an outbreak of eczema wherever the X-rays had contacted the body. This dark-red rash caused severe irritation. She then lay sleepless in bed for months. Finally, her husband produced an ointment which cured the eczema, but it was soon followed by bronchitis and shingles. She had continual relapses until 1951. All this time the bowel movements had been very painful; the constipation would not yield to treatment, and the intestine was ulcerated. Her chronic headache and attacks of dizziness still persisted.

Shortly before Christmas, 1951, the old gnawing pains began again in the abdomen. Frau Lingenfelder clearly understood what this portended and began the new year in a hopeless frame of mind.

Deliverance was on the way, however. Are Waerland came to lecture in Munich. She dragged herself painfully to the hall and heard with amazement not only of a new biological system of nutrition but also of its wonderful effects on widely different diseases. The lecture made a deep impression on her mind, and she went home resolved to alter the family diet.

After only a few days Frau Lingenfelder began to notice a change in her own condition and, as time went on, one symptom after another disappeared. Natural bowel movements began the good work of clearing out the toxins, and she lost the heavy sense of weariness. Her infected tonsils cleared up and the arthritic pains left her knees. The heart was relieved and her skin grew supple and youthful. She was soon able to cope with physical and mental efforts which had previously been impossible. After having been an invalid for eight years, she was finally able to join in outdoor pursuits, especially her favorite sport of swimming. The greatest miracle was that the bowel was completely healed.

Frau B., also German, was another desperate case who regained her health through the Waerland therapy. Here again, the disease had been brought on through long-standing constipation due to a wrong way of living and unnatural, unbiological diet. For a long time Frau B. had only two or three evacuations per week. Menstrual disturbances had been treated with hormone injections and, after the birth of her second child, corrective treatment of the pelvis had been necessary. She suffered from chronic headache, was always tired, and had rheumatic pains.

One day she discovered a hardening of the right breast and went to a doctor who advised immediate removal of the breast. This was done a few days later, but the operation proved not to have been comprehensive enough. Later, all the lymphatic glands in the armpit had to be cut away. A series of X-ray treatments—twenty radiations in all—were given. The right arm was now completely useless and swelled alarmingly on the slightest movement. Her general condition grew much worse and she had severe heart attacks.

About nine months after the breast amputation, at Christmas, 1950, she began to study our literature and acted on it. After only a few days on the new diet the bowels functioned better and in ten days the headache had gone. A swelling in the left hip gradually grew smaller and disappeared. These results were obtained through regular fasts under our supervision, and the patient finally made a complete recovery. She said she felt "born again" and was full of vitality and the joy of living such as she had never known before.

The cases of Frau Lingenfelder and Frau B. are sufficient to show what can be done by natural methods even for cancer sufferers. Many more stories of remarkable cures are to be found in the back numbers of the *Waerland Monthly Magazine,* published in Sweden.*

One interesting case was that of a man (A.M.), suffering from spinal cancer. He underwent eight operations for tumors, and part of the lower spine was removed. The condition was malignant at all the operations except the last, when the surgeons expressed surprise on finding that the tumor was benign. This operation was performed after the patient had been for a considerable time on a lacto-vegetarian diet.

Dr. Jonas Kristjansson, a well-known Icelandic surgeon, took a keen interest in Waerland's work from the very beginning. He not only built up his own health by a change of diet but also treated his patients according to Waerland principles, with excellent results. As District Medical Officer for a large area, he was known as "the friend of the hopeless." The desperately sick turned to him when no one else could do anything for them, and he was often able to help them find the way back to health. Here is one of the cases he told me about:

* The author has these available at her home in Sweden.

A patient came to him, a woman with large cancerous swellings in both breasts. The doctors had been unable to help her and had finally declared her incurable, the disease having gone too far to operate. She came to Dr. Kristjansson, not to be cured, for she had given up all hope of that, but to learn from him how to arrange her diet for the remainder of her life so as to avoid, if possible, the terrible pain before the end.

Dr. Kristjansson advised her to live exclusively on rawkost and milk. Even her potatoes were to be eaten *raw*.

When the woman left him, the doctor expected never to see her again but, to his amazement, she came back after ten months glowing with health and gratitude. An examination proved that the growths had completely disappeared. A blood test revealed that her previously very low hemoglobin was now 100%. Her general condition was excellent.

Diet and treatment for cancer

This disease, which in civilized man usually appears after the age of forty, is a typical degenerative disease, caused largely by a faulty diet and manner of living.

All foods which have been treated chemically, or through cooking and sterilizing have been robbed of their minerals and vitamins, besides all animal proteins in the form of meat, fish, and eggs, are factors which lead to the outbreak of cancer. They all contain cholesterol, which is found to excess in the blood of certain types of cancer patients.

Since cancer never breaks out before the poisoning and disorganization of the body have reached a certain degree, it is clear that preventive treatment is of the utmost importance. If the disease has already broken out, the first thing to be done is to clear away all impurities and toxins. In acute cases this can gradually be achieved by fasting. Other important factors to be observed are daily exercise in the fresh air, baths, and care of the skin.

In many cases fasting is the surest way to health for the cancer patient. A short fast of a week is the first step. This is followed by a week of a highly alkaline diet which includes two rawkost meals daily. Sweet milk and milk products are to be avoided and bread is cut down to a minimum, only bread baked with sourdough* being allowed. After a week, the second fasting period of two weeks is introduced and this time is followed by two weeks on the alkaline diet. After a further three-weeks' fast, followed by three weeks of the diet, the final, long fast of four weeks begins. If the disease has advanced so far that it cannot be checked, it is at least possible, by fasting, to minimize the indescribable agony that cancer patients often endure before deliverance comes and the martyred body finds rest.

There are various homeopathic preparations which have been used with some success in treating cancerous diseases, especially mistletoe, and in Germany I have, in a few cases, used a biologic preparation named "plantalact." But no remedies are of any avail whatsoever unless the pa-

* '*Surdeg*' (sourdough): a piece of dough saved from the previous baking. (See p. 207.)

tient has the right diet, and then only when it is backed up by cleansing treatment and fasting.

The most important factor, the prerequisite in fact, for the success of any physical treatment, including fasting, is the patient's own attitude to his condition, his courage, his will to live and his inherent energy.

Composition of diet

On waking: Morning drink. Potato or vegetable decoction. Add linseed and bran as required. (See p. 199.)

Breakfast: Sour milk and fruit. According to taste the milk may be topped with bran, linseed, and milk sugar, or powdered rose hips and nettles.

Midmorning: Herb tea.

Lunch: All kinds of raw vegetables; as much onion and garlic as the patient can tolerate; potatoes, cooked and raw; sour milk; a slice of leavened bread. Raw vegetable juices; two dessertspoonfuls of cold-pressed oil; sauerkraut (unsalted). Cabbage juice is particularly valuable for cancer patients but must be diluted with half vegetable broth.

Midafternoon: Herb tea.

Supper: The same as lunch.

10 / *Diabetes*

Diabetes in its various forms is one of the very widespread "diseases of civilization." It is a functional disease, caused by failure of the insulin-producing cells of the pancreas. Without insulin the body is unable to regulate the conversion of the starch of carbohydrates into blood sugar, the only form in which it can be assimilated and become "fuel" for the body. This is one of the most delicately balanced processes of the human organism, and when it is disturbed the effects are very serious and difficult to correct. When sugar is found in abnormal quantities in the blood and urine, it is a sign that the islets of Langerhans in the pancreas have become overloaded or poisoned and that they are unable to deal with the amount of starch normally contained in the diet.

This is an advanced stage of the disease at which it is generally regarded by academic medicine as incurable. To restore the balance, insulin secretions from the bodies of animals are injected, which enable the patient to carry on a more or less normal life, within certain limitations, as long as the injections are regularly kept up. Meanwhile, the cells whose job it is to produce the insulin, being no longer called upon to do so, become superfluous, and they atrophy beyond repair.

When diabetes has been diagnosed, the patient is usually admitted into a hospital for tests to be made determining the dosage of insulin required to enable him to carry on life on an ordinary "civilized" diet.

Logical reasoning must lead to the view that this is entirely wrong!

The most natural thing to do would be to reduce the starch content in the daily dietary and carefully introduce a diet that would place the least possible burden on the pancreas, thus giving it a chance to recover. This is the aim of the Waerland treatment and it must be said that, as long as no external insulin is introduced, the cells can usually be regenerated in a surprisingly short time.

Unfortunately, diabetes is one of the diseases more difficult to cure in children than in adults. In my experience it is practically impossible to cure a young child of diabetes if insulin has been used for any length of time. When the insulin-producing cells have become weakened or poisoned and their function is replaced by secretions from animals, their development is arrested and they atrophy altogether.

Most of the young children who have come under my care have had insulin for some time, and therefore it has not been possible to arrest the disease. On the other hand, if the children had had no insulin or only for a short time, we had wonderful results. Children aged about ten years *who had only been on insulin for a short period* responded readily and very good results were obtained.

According to unanimous accounts from parents, diabetic children are given exactly the same food as others in our Swedish hospitals. If this actually is the case, a child whose insulin-producing cells have broken down and are no longer able to function receives an overdose of precisely the kind of foods which encourage the disease, with carbohydrates at every meal and sweets and chocolates allowed between meals. Large doses of insulin are, naturally, required to cope with this diet. Nothing is more unnatural or unreasonable than to give starch in its various forms to diabetics and, at the same time, inject larger and larger doses of insulin to deal with it.

It would seem that the orthodox mind finds it quite natural to introduce into the organism those secretions which it should itself produce. But these methods of treatment seem to us to be at cross purposes with the laws of nature and, therefore, not so likely to meet with success as a method which not only co-operates with nature but also calls in all the wealth of natural forces to help restore the lost balance and weakened cells of the pancreas.

If, immediately on discovering diabetes in a child, a carefully planned diet were introduced, avoiding as far as possible all foods which put a strain on the insulin-producing cells, it would be found that in practically every case a rapid improvement—in many cases complete recovery—would ensue. The same applies, of course, to adult diabetics, but it must be emphasized that anyone who has had diabetes will always have to observe great moderation with regard to starchy foods, even after recovery, in order not to overstrain the cells again. Almost every human body has a weak spot, and this must be faced and taken into account. We each have different hereditary tendencies and it is important for our health that we should realize our limitations and arrange our lives accordingly.

The most important thing one can do for a patient is to teach him to know his own body, with all its disabilities and weaknesses, so that he can become his own physician. What a joy it is when this succeeds and one can say to him: "Now you can take the care of your health into your own hands because there is nobody in the world who understands it better than you do yourself." These are the patients who have no relapses and who attain lasting health.

Young diabetic patients, especially those in their teens, need a great deal of patience and endurance if they have had insulin injections for some time, in order to achieve lasting results. If they have not had insulin, the improvement is surprisingly rapid. As a rule, diabetes is more easily cured the older the patient is.

Small children are more difficult to treat because they cannot fast under the age of twelve, and fasting is the best of all remedies. It is a great mistake to think that a diabetic cannot fast on raw juices from root vegetables because of the sugar they contain. On the contrary, this natural sugar, being quite different from the industrialized, dead sugar and even from the fruit sugar in dried fruits and some sweet fresh fruits (such as bananas and pears), can be beneficially assimilated by the diabetic organism.

Fasting for a diabetic, and also his diet, must be carefully arranged for each individual in relation to the quantity of sugar and acids in his blood and urine. The diet should consist almost exclusively of raw vegetables with a little sour milk and acid fruits, a little butter and oil and diabetic—or rheumatic—bread. Where an excess of acids is found, he should have more potatoes. If the heightened sugar content is the main symptom, the quantity of potatoes should be reduced and other raw vegetables increased.

Whether a patient fasts or not, he must drink *beanskin* (*Phaseolus*) *tea* four times a day, two cups for an adult and one cup for a child each time. Beanskin tea is a substitute for insulin but does not, like animal insulin, prevent the regeneration of the insulin-producing cells. Teas and herbal drugs obtained from the vegetable kingdom are better than allopathic medicines for strengthening our various organs and stimulating them to better functioning. It is important to give the healing juices of living plants in their natural composition so that they do not disturb the balance of our physical economy. If this balance is upset by the intake of chemical, synthetically produced preparations, it is bad, even if important substances such as vitamins and hormones are being introduced. Our organism is such a finely balanced mechanism that every excess of any substance, however vital, causes some disturbance of its functioning which may have detrimental effects.

Instructions for taking beanskin tea and fasting for diabetic patients will be found at the end of this chapter, also the basic guide for their dietary. It is of the greatest importance that the vegetables included in the daily food of a diabetic contain precisely those elements which are important to the functioning of the insulin-producing cells. The vegetables which are richest in these elements are cucumber, celery, celeriac, Jerusalem artichokes, and onions. Tender young nettles and dandelion leaves are very beneficial. The nettles may be lightly boiled, stewed, or infused as tea, and the dandelion leaves eaten as salad or made into tea. In general, teas made from herbs and leaves should not be too strong, but dandelions and nettles are the exception to this rule. The *raw* juices of dandelion leaves and nettles, diluted with an equal quantity of potato water, are excellent.

It is absolutely essential, in treating diabetics, to cleanse the intestine by enemas and colonic irrigation.

Herr M., born in 1917, came to us at Kiholm in the summer of 1953, having had diabetes for five years. When he arrived, his acidity was very high and our doctor found his condition so serious that he urged us to send him to a hospital. He considered that we should not take the responsibility of such a serious and far-advanced case. But I begged to be allowed at least to make an attempt to save the young man, for I could well imagine the kind of treatment that he would have in a hospital and the effect it would have on the remainder of his life. The percentage of sugar in the blood and urine was not high—2% urine sugar and 0.220 blood sugar. It was the acids which were alarmingly high. On August 18 the Gerhard test showed plus 2 and the Legal test plus 3.

Herr M. was put on a special fast, adapted to the high percentage of acids. After only a couple of days the urine sugar had gone down to 0.160, Gerhard to plus 1, and

Legal to plus 2. On August 26 the blood sugar was normal, the urine sugar 0.24, and the acids almost gone. After twelve days' fasting there were no more acids and the urine sugar was normal. The patient's general condition was excellent. He was able to begin the special modified-sugar diet and it suited him well.

K.E. was a man of forty who was sent to Kiholm to be treated for diabetes by the chief medical officer in his home town. He had very high acidity and his blood sugar was 0.305. Happily he had been having insulin for only three months and we were able to stop it and put him on a fast at once. After one week he had no more acids, the urine was free from sugar, and the blood sugar had gone down to 0.145. A month later he left Kiholm, fully recovered.

This cannot be done in cases where the patient has been on insulin for a long time. It can certainly be reduced to about half the dosage as soon as the patient goes on to a diet from which starches have been reduced to a minimum and which contains elements that will revive and build up the insulin cells, but the injections must be continued until the sugar and acids have diminished and are sufficiently under control for it to be left off without risk. Such cases are very protracted, as the fast cannot be begun as long as the patient is having insulin.

The reason for this is that in many obstinate cases the sugar disappears during a fast but returns as soon as the patient begins to eat. It is therefore necessary to renew the fasting several times, with intervals, until the improvement has advanced so far that the patient is able to benefit from his specially adapted diet without the recurrence of any trace of sugar or acids. The blood and urine of a diabetic must be continually checked, tests being made twice a week during treatment and, even after recovery, an occasional check. The goal to be aimed at is, of course, that he will eventually be able to amplify his diet, but this must not be done without careful checking.

H.S. was an old lady from Gothenburg. She had been a diabetic for eight years, following pneumonia. Guided by a sound instinct, she had refused to have insulin and we were able to start her on a fast at once. On arrival at Kiholm her blood sugar was 0.375. After only three days of fasting it had gone down to 0.145, where it remained even after the fast was broken.

Similar results have been achieved in many cases with elderly people.

W.J., a man of sixty, came to Elmau, our first sanatorium in Germany, seeking a cure for long-standing diabetes. He had had up to 5.9% of urine sugar. After a stay of one month he was completely cured.

E.J., born in 1915, had diabetes after pneumonia and had been in bed for several months. To begin with, he was given twelve units of insulin, but this was increased more and more until on his arrival at Kiholm he was having forty units daily. This patient stayed with us only two and a half weeks but achieved normal sugar percentage in that time. When he went home he was perfectly well.

Now, many of our opponents argue that such a rapid change cannot possibly mean a cure of the disease. They say that we have only temporarily eliminated the symptoms by removing the starch from the patient's food, and that if he were to go back to an ordinary civilized diet the quantity of sugar in blood and urine would again increase. Consequently, the patient is not well. So they say.

Let me here ask one question: if a diabetic patient, by means of a well-balanced natural diet, succeeds in eliminating the pathological quantity of sugar in his blood and urine while, at the same time, his general condition steadily improves, is it not then illogical to regard him as ill? Can it not legitimately be said that the disease has been cured?

A certain organic weakness of the insulin-producing cells not unnaturally remains for some time, but the fact that they are unable to stand up to a diet which is unnatural and undermining is not necessarily a sign of bad health.

Treatment of diabetes

The most important measure is, at first, a thorough internal cleansing. Therefore diabetics must have an enema night and morning until some improvement is evident, and after that in the evening only. When the natural rhythm of bowel evacuation has become established (three to four movements daily), the enemas are stopped. If the bowel does not function regularly, the patient changes to the small, cool enemas of a pint of water. (See instructions for enemas, p. 198.)

As already pointed out, the invalid must be very careful in the choice of diet and avoid all foods which contain starch which, in the body, is converted into sugar. On changing over to the Waerland diet the patient must do so only under the supervision of a doctor. His food should consist mainly of sour milk, raw fruit, and raw vegetables. To begin with, until the sugar content in the blood and urine has gone down, he may not eat potatoes or diabetic bread except in very small quantities. On changing over to this diet, the daily dose of insulin must immediately be reduced by at least one third to one half. Afterward the dose is reduced gradually as the sugar content diminishes. If the patient carefully follows the directions for a reduced sugar diet, if he drinks his beanskin tea regularly three to four times a day and attends to the internal cleansing, progressive improvement begins as a rule very soon. By degrees the quantity of starch in the food may be increased (potatoes and cereals) until the patient is fully recovered and able to eat the ordinary Waerland diet.

Treatment of diabetic patients who have not had insulin

In these cases a fast must be started at once, provided that heart, kidneys, lungs, and thyroid gland are still functioning fairly satisfactorily. Should any of these organs be so far impaired that a full fast is impossible, a kind of semi-fast must be worked out to suit the patient.

The length of the fast varies with the individual. As soon as the sugar content in the blood and urine has become normal and there is no excess of acids, the patient continues the fast for only a few days and then carefully changes over to the special low-sugar diet. It often happens that all counts become normal after even a very short fast. During the fast an enema is, of course, given night and morning. *Patients who have to take insulin* must not fast, but begin straight away on the low-sugar diet.

Directions for fasting

The patient must drink from 2 to 2½ quarts daily. *On waking, in the forenoon, in the afternoon, and perhaps also in the evening* he drinks two cups of beanskin tea, i.e., six to eight cups altogether.

For breakfast, lunch, and dinner he has raw juice from green leaves (¼ of raw juice to ¾ of potato water or vegetable broth) *OR* raw juices from root vegetables (diluted by ⅓ to ¼ of potato water or vegetable broth). The best juices are from celeriac, cucumber, and Jerusalem artichokes.

After the fast the enemas are discontinued except when required, and then it should be in the evening, shortly after dinner. The small, cool enemas are best, as these can be continued indefinitely without detriment.

Diet for diabetic patients

On waking, Midmorning & Afternoon: Beanskin tea, for adults two cups each time; children one cup. To make the drink more palatable for children, the juice of an orange may be added. (For preparation of beanskin tea, see p. 195.)

Breakfast: Sour milk topped with bran, linseed and, perhaps, dried powdered nettles or rose hips. Fruit (oranges or not-too-sweet apples are best). Sweet fruit, such as pears, bananas, grapes, and sweet dried fruits such as figs, dates, raisins, and prunes are prohibited.

Lunch: All kinds of raw vegetables with, especially, large quantities of celery or celeriac, cucumber, artichokes, and onions. Raw juices, including, in summer, the juice of nettle and dandelion leaves. Chopped as salad or stewed, both these plants are beneficial. Potatoes, butter, cold-pressed oil, diabetic bread. No cheese except cottage cheese (preparation p. 197). A glass of sour milk. The quantity of potatoes must vary: if the patient has a high acid count he takes more potatoes, i.e., two or three medium-size ones. If the abnormal sugar content in blood and urine is the primary symptom, he takes very little potato.

Dinner: Same as lunch.

Prohibited: All ordinary bread, kruska, molino and all cereals and foods containing sugar.

Beanskin tea is a natural substitute for insulin. The skin of the pods of green beans* and the thin membrane around the beans themselves are very rich in silicic acid and another substance which is closely related to insulin. They are therefore extremely beneficial in diabetes and also rheumatism and arthritis. One cup of beanskin tea is equal to at least one unit of insulin. The sugar content in blood and urine is reduced, and the patient's ability to

* *Phaseolus:* French, or kidney, bean. Dried beanskin is available in some European drugstores.

tolerate starchy foods is increased. The acids are also reduced. The quantity of urine increases, the kidneys excrete more uric acid while the content of uric acid in the blood is reduced. Inflammation in the veins and eczema, which often occur in diabetics, are also cured by beanskin tea.

Cucumber contains an enzyme needed by the cells in order to produce insulin. *Celery* and *Celeriac* are rich in alkaline salts and vital substances which have a beneficial effect in diabetes. It also contains starch and sugar in a form assimilable by diabetics. Celeriac is not only good for the pancreas and its insulin-producing cells but for all the glands of our body and our nerves and for the female organs. Like cucumber and the carrot, it is an excellent remedy for rheumatism, kidney troubles, and gallstones. *The Onion* contains certain hormones beneficial in diabetes.

11 / *Eczema and psoriasis*

Psoriasis is usually regarded as incurable, but we have found that most cases yield to dietetic treatment.

Eczema and psoriasis are the result of excessive accumulations of waste products and residues. The body is trying to eliminate through the skin these surplus impurities which the other organs have not been able to throw out. It is against the laws of nature and quite wrong to try to suppress the eruptions by means of ointments and medications. Suppressive treatment of this kind does not often succeed, but when it does, the apparent cure can only be regarded as a doubtful service to the body. For eruptions of the skin, and boils, are a typical sign that the other organs of elimination are not able to rid the body of the harmful substances collected in the tissues. All the toxins and waste substances which can find no other way out have to be thrown out via the skin. If this cleansing process is stopped, the body will be further poisoned and serious organic disturbances will occur.

The most important thing in dealing with these diseases is, of course, to assist the eliminative processes in every way by fasting, enemas, and colonic irrigation. In acute cases of psoriasis, improvement is noticeable only during the fasts, the condition remaining static during the intervals when the patient is again eating. Thus, the cure consists of a series of fasts with intervals during which the patient has the Waerland diet specially adapted for these cases, as a result of many years of experimentation and experience.

Treatment of psoriasis and eczema

As already stated, fasting is the most important feature of the treatment of these diseases. The patients usually fast on raw juices (see p. 200), but in certain cases fasting on water only has to be resorted to for a short time. In obstinate cases the fast will have to be repeated at intervals. The pauses between the fasts are shorter or longer, depending upon how quickly the patient regains normal weight. It is not essential for all the lost weight to be made up, but before each new period of fasting the patient must be in good condition generally.

During the fasts no physical treatment is given, except, of course, the enema morning and evening, but when the fast is over the patients have a warm soda bath (see p. 202) twice a week. They do not need to perspire, either in the bath or afterward, as the rheumatic patients do. The bath is intended merely to soften and remove the scabs. Two pounds of soda are used for each bath, and the patient lies in it for ten minutes. Those suffering from "weeping" eczema should not take baths or wash with water. The skin must be washed daily with a decoction of camomile or horsetail. If the bowel does not begin to act spontaneously, an enema should be given on the evening of the second day after breaking the fast (not before). As long as the bowel rhythm is not established, the evening enema should be continued, preferably the small, cool one of a pint of lukewarm water.

Diet for eczema and psoriasis patients

On waking: Morning drink—vegetable broth in which two tablespoonfuls each of linseed and bran have been steeped overnight. A pint of this for each person is warmed up in the morning. Stir to keep the bran afloat, and drink everything!

Breakfast: Sour milk topped with bran and linseed, or powdered rose hips or nettles, or other green vitamins. Carrot juice. In slighter cases, acid fruit.

Midmorning & Afternoon: Herb tea, preferably horsetail or camomile.

Lunch: All kinds of raw vegetables (onions to be avoided in most cases). Raw juices. As much potato as desired, sour milk, cottage cheese and rheumatic bread (recipe p. 195).

Dinner: The same as lunch or, for a change, our potato porridge (recipe p. 205) with sour milk and bran, rheumatic bread, and cottage cheese.

Forbidden: Everything that contains sugar, salt, or fat (except milk). Also kruska, molino, and ordinary bread. Also, of course, sweet dried fruit and all sweet fresh fruit.

There are certain acute cases in which no animal protein in any form can be tolerated. In these cases the sour milk must be omitted and protein obtained in soya beans (cooked or raw; if raw, they should be sprouted: see p. 208).

It is important to give the patient vitamin B, preferably in the form of brewer's yeast. There are also various preparations on the market abroad, such as Vitamin F.99, which have proved helpful in these cases.

Large numbers of hopeless psoriasis cases have in this way been completely cured both at Kiholm and at the various sanatoria I have worked in abroad. Here are a few typical cases.

S.S., whom I treated in the autumn of 1950 at Kiholm, was a very bad case. He was a man of about forty who had suffered from psoriasis for eight years. His case had long before been pronounced incurable. Since 1942 he had been wandering from one hospital to another. In 1946 arthritis had set in. All his joints were affected; he could move only with great difficulty and had much pain. The whole of his skin from the soles of his feet to the crown of his head was covered with bluish-red, scaly and weeping scurf. Mattery boils had come out all over his body.

He stayed at Kiholm for four months and during that time he fasted sixty days in periods of ten days, with ten-day intervals. Improvement began after the first fast. When he left, the patient had a fine, delicate skin, as rosy and soft as a baby's. Only on the bridge of his nose there remained a small patch and a few small boils on his hands.

Mrs. K.B., from Gothenburg, was another remarkable case. She was twenty-four and had had eczema since she was seven. Most of the time she had unbearable itching. Treatment in hospitals had given her no relief. The eczema was "weeping" and the itching had become worse, so that when she arrived at Kiholm she was desperate. She could not sleep and her life was nothing but a martyrdom. Her nerves were strained to the breaking point.

Mrs. B. had intended to stay at Kiholm for four weeks to have a thorough course of treatment. But as she had already tried so many treatments, she had not much hope that this new experiment would help. For seventeen years she had been seeking a cure, trying all the methods of traditional medicine. She began her fasting and cleansing treatment with small expectations.

Her astonishment when the itching stopped after only five days' fasting may be imagined, and when the eczema had gone after twelve days it was a miracle to all who witnessed it.

Each organism has its individual ability to react to treatment, but this is its own secret. Therefore it is never possible to say *how soon* the improvement will become evident or *when* the disrupted balance in the body will be restored. There may be very severe cases where the recuperative forces of the body are still strong. In such cases inexplicable miracles of swift healing may occur. On the other hand, there are apparently slight cases for which one expects a rapid recovery, which prove unexpectedly obstinate and slow. Even the most sensitive instruments science can invent can never penetrate the hidden processes of the living cells which make up our organism. We can never measure, or weigh, that most important of all health-building factors—the Life Force, the concealed source of health within each of us.

Ultimately, it is upon this Force that our recuperative powers depend. They are not governed solely by the circumstances of the body but, also, by those of the mind. There are delicate people with fragile bodies who seem as if a puff of wind would be sufficient to put out the flame of life in them, but who are able to fulfill apparently impossible tasks and survive the most terrible illnesses without breaking up. From inexhaustible streams of life, unknown to us, they draw their strength, and where the physically strong go under, they emerge victorious from their suffering.

Mrs. B. did not, after all, stay at Kiholm as long as she had expected. After sixteen days she declared that she now felt so well that she would like to go home.

One would have thought that such a rapid recovery could not be lasting. But it held, and during the years that have passed I have had only good accounts from the patient.

Sven I., a man of fifty, was another of our eczema patients at Kiholm. He had been suffering for the past four years from weeping sores all over his body, for which he had not been able to find relief, although he had consulted many doctors.

His wife told me in a letter how he had suffered ever since he had developed eczema twenty years before. This had slowly spread over the body, coming and going periodically, but for the last four years there had been no remission. Mr. I. had consulted the best specialists he could find and had been in various hospitals, all without result. He had now been advised to go into the hospital again. Owing to the agony of his illness he had become completely apathetic, having lost all will power and all hope.

He came to Kiholm as a result of persuasion by his wife and, somewhat skeptically, submitted to our treatment. He, too, experienced the miracle of regeneration through fasting and inward cleansing. As soon as the poisons had been cleared, the eczema and maddening itching disappeared. At last the healing forces in his own body had been assisted in their work, the forces which are always ready to heal and repair all damage and deficiency for us, if only we co-operate. We are all too prone to poison our blood and our organs with the residues of unsuitable food, injurious luxuries, and medications.

Mr. I. went home after three weeks, a new man, with only a few insignificant traces left of his former eczema but with a new will-to-live and the ability to enjoy life once more.

These cases clearly show that skin diseases of the nature of eczema and psoriasis are due to inner filth and will yield to properly conducted fasting and internal cleansing.

12 / *Diseases of the stomach and intestines; ulcers*

Little did I ever imagine, during the thirty-five years of my apparently incurable colitis, which baffled the most famous specialists in Europe, that I should one day be well and be able to lead countless other sufferers along the road to health.

My faith in doctors was blind. I never reflected on the fact that they, too, could be ill and often, indeed, suffered from stomach and intestinal troubles themselves. They were surrounded by a sort of halo, and I was convinced that no one would be able to help me if the doctors could not do so. But then the miracle happened!

As my digestive organs were in such a bad state, it seemed at first impossible for me to tolerate the new diet. But how thankful I am now that I had so many obstacles to overcome and that my intestinal trouble was so severe. For I was given the opportunity of finding out through my own experience just how these hopeless cases can be cured.

The first essential for health and for curing the many ills that assail our bodies is that our digestive organs be in good condition. If they are weak and degenerated, an apparently insuperable obstacle is set up which we have to overcome before any headway can be made. It is an unfortunate fact that in this age of civilization, the stomach and intestines of a large majority of people have become slack, dilated, and dropped and are consequently no longer able to deal with a diet consisting of health-giving foods containing roughage in the form of whole grains, raw green vegetables, and roots.

The digestive glands, too, are often out of order, so that a deficiency or a surplus of hydrochloric acid and other digestive juices occurs. The acid-forming nature of present-day diet is largely to blame for the prevalence of gastric or duodenal ulcers, because the corrosive action of too much hydrochloric acid destroys the delicate mucous membrane of the stomach. Insufficient mastication, the rush and worry of modern life with consequent nervous tension and anxiety also interfere with the functions of the digestive organs and cause serious disturbances.

Most people suffering from gastric ulcers are depressed and nervous. They often develop illusions, neuroses, and a deficiency of vitamin B. It is not to be wondered at that the nervous system is affected when the whole organism is undernourished and weakened owing to the inability of the digestive organs to assimilate the food.

In spite of the usually emaciated and anemic condition of a gastric-ulcer patient, it is entirely wrong to try to fatten him up with "nourishing" food. It is the most disastrous thing one can do. The shortest and indeed the only way back to health, is by fasting. But not on any account a fast on water only, which would increase the excessive acidity. Nor is the usual fast on raw root-vegetable juices suitable here. Although carrot juice has great healing properties, it cannot be tolerated in large quantities by gastric-ulcer patients. We have, therefore, evolved a drink which is wonderfully healing and at the same time contains plenty of minerals and is highly alkaline. Supplemented by carrot juice *in small quantities,* it works wonders in all stomach and intestinal disorders caused by irritated, ulcerated mucous membranes. In order to reduce the surplus of acids still further, occasional tablespoonfuls of raw potato juice may be given.

The decoction is made from potatoes, linseed, and wheat bran according to the following recipe (also on p. 198).

Recipe for a decoction for gastric ulcers

Soak 3 tablespoonfuls of whole linseed (flaxseed) and 6 tablespoonfuls of wheat bran overnight in 3 pints of hot water. In the morning, boil for 20 to 30 minutes until thick and slimy, from time to time thinning it down with a little water. Wash and cut into slices 1 lb. of raw potatoes, *with the skin,* and boil for about 20 minutes in 3 pints of water. This may also be diluted if it gets too thick. Strain both decoctions through a sieve, mix together while still hot, and stand to cool. Care must be taken not to let it go sour.

Composition of diet for gastric-ulcer patients

For the first ten days the patient fasts on the ulcer decoction, taking 200 grams (4/5 cupful) of the decoction plus

100 grams of carrot juice (⅖ cup) every two hours, from 7:00 or 8:00 in the morning until 7:00 or 8:00 in the evening—that is: seven times daily. If at first he is unable to tolerate so much carrot juice, a very small quantity should be tried and gradually increased to the full amount, keeping the total quantity of fluid always at 300 grams (1⅕ cups) of fluid.

An enema is given morning and evening, first a small one of a pint, expelled immediately, and then a quart. Both are given with tepid water for gastric-ulcer patients, and with the addition of camomile decoction or kaolin if the bowel is ulcerated.

The fast should be broken with a little sour milk *for breakfast on the eleventh day.*

For lunch and dinner, boiled potatoes, peeled and mashed, with a little mild sour milk as dressing.

Early morning, midmorning, and afternoon, also in the evening if desired, two cups of the decoction.

Both food and drink should be slowly insalivated and well chewed. Always rest after eating.

On the second day after the fast has been broken, the following dietary should be started and maintained for ten days:

On waking, midmorning & afternoon: Decoction with added carrot juice.

Breakfast: Mild sour milk with carrot juice (½ glass).

Lunch: Potatoes peeled and mashed; the same quantity of carrot juice as at breakfast; mild sour milk.

Dinner: Potatoes, peeled and mashed; boiled carrots; a glass of half milk and half water. Wheat rusks.

At the end of this period of 21 days a little cottage cheese may be taken.

After about three weeks the *breakfast* may be augmented by milk sugar (on the sour milk) and, possibly, powdered nettles and a finely grated sweet apple without the skin. *To the lunch* may be added a little finely grated carrot, tender lettuce, or endive. The patient must cautiously feel his way and never begin with more than one new item at the same time, to make sure that this particular thing suits him. Small quantities of cold-pressed oils may now be introduced (in cases of intestinal ulcers these may be begun sooner), and cooked spinach may be added to the lunch with advantage also dandelion or nettle juice diluted with potato water (⅓ juice-⅔ potato water). *Dinner* may be varied by a meal of potato porridge with apple sauce (not too much sweetened), wholemeal rusks, and undiluted milk.

After four weeks the menu may be considerably augmented. Butter (which in intestinal cases may be introduced after three weeks) may now be taken. Molino (recipe p. 204) may serve as an alternative to potato porridge; and with the vegetable meal, various raw salads (vegetable) and grated roots (especially beets and celery), graham bread and whey cheese.*

Forbidden foods are very coarse bread, kruska, and

* Norwegian *gjetost* or *geitost* is whey cheese. There are two kinds available in some of the larger metropolitan areas of America and in places where there are many Scandinavians: the *ekte*, made of the whey of goat's milk only, and the regular, made of the whey of both goat's and cow's milk. As with some other foods, it may take more than one taste of gjetost to develop a liking for it.

onions. These must not be even tried until several months after the patient's complete recovery.

It is important to treat every case with the utmost individual attention.

Of all the numerous cases I have treated in this way in the course of many years, I can recall only two in which the patient had a relapse. In both cases it was due to a departure from the prescribed diet. People who have been seriously ill and have regained their health through our therapy can seldom revert to their former ways of eating and living without bringing on the old symptoms again.

The following case is typical of what should *not* be done. It illustrates the academic view of the problem and is very enlightening:

Herr B. came for treatment to one of our larger sanatoria in Switzerland, at which I was being assisted by a doctor who was greatly interested in our principles but had not yet fully accepted our view of the problem of disease.

For over twenty years Herr B. had been suffering from bleeding gastric ulcers with repeated vomiting of blood. Having several years previously changed over to the Waerland diet, he had managed to carry on, in spite of strenuous manual work. Unfortunately, however, he had not understood how to adapt the diet to the gastric ulcer and had now come to me to get the better of his complaint and try to heal the ulcers.

Thanks to the diet, his blood was in good condition, but he was very thin. The doctor declared at once that the first thing to do was to give him a nourishing diet with butter and cream. It cost me incredible effort to convince him that the only way to get a satisfactory result was through fasting.

The patient himself was full of confidence and entrusted himself to my care for the first ten days of fasting on the decoction, with enemas night and morning. During this period the healing process would advance sufficiently for him to go on to the next stage, on the eleventh day, i.e., to boiled potatoes, boiled carrots, mild sour milk, and carrot juice. After a further ten days we would go further to the next stage of the healing diet.

A certain loss of weight during a fast is inevitable, but it is relatively unimportant, since no increase in weight *can* be achieved until the ulcer has healed and the patient is again able to assimilate his food. It is, therefore, unnecessary and harmful to worry the patient by frequent weighing and anxious, negative comments when what he most needs is to be calm and peaceful. But in this case the patient's weight was checked daily and he was made to feel unduly anxious. In spite of this the healing went on quickly and well during the fast; he felt stronger and the pains ceased altogether. After the fast was broken the improvement went on apace, and it was touching to see the patient's joy. In spite of—or, more accurately, thanks to—the simple, moderate diet, he began to gain weight.

At this point the doctor began to take an energetic hand in the proceedings. When the patient consulted him, he advised him to eat large portions and to begin taking butter and cream. All my warnings were now in vain. The newly regained health had brought with it an enormous appetite and the patient, who had felt his strength increasing day by day, became too venturesome. At the same time we had unfortunately had a consignment of artificially fertilized and sprayed potatoes, which the staff and many of the guests refused to eat, but which our ulcer patient, with his newly aroused appetite, ate indiscriminately in large quantities. The consequences were not slow in coming: the ulcer broke again.

At this point I was called away on urgent duties in another country. Reluctantly, I had to leave the patient in the doctor's hands and never saw him again.

The results of other cases we have treated have been just as successful as this one was tragic in its outcome. The following are some of those recorded in my card index. They show that, even in cases where hope has been abandoned by the doctors, there is still hope of improvement, often complete recovery. It is a matter of cautiously and consistently supporting the recuperative faculty of the body.

This means trying to find the foods which the digestive organs are able to make use of, so that the rebuilding of the organism may begin. Needless to say, this diet must be as complete as possible, simple and scanty though it has to be. We have treated and cured cases where the digestive organs could hardly assimilate any food at all. One of the most severe was that of Mrs. M.

The patient, an elderly lady, had come by ambulance the long journey from Kleines Walsertal in Austria to

Sonnenhof, Thun (Switzerland) to seek my help. For many years she had had gastric ulcers, with constantly recurrent bleeding, and cancer was suspected. Eighteen days before she came to us she had had a violent attack and vomited blood. Her heart was badly affected and she was unable to assimilate any food or drink. The doctor who was called in wished her to go into the hospital at once and have blood transfusions to try to save her life. Even I, who hardly ever give up hope, felt that her case was desperate and agreed with him. Mrs. M. was like a mummy, emaciated, with parchmentlike skin.

But the seventy-year-old lady refused to leave Sonnenhof. We had to let her stay. Happily, her daughter had come with her and was a great help to me. The patient still was unable to assimilate any food. Where could we find a starting point from which we could commence the work of rehabilitation? Even the ulcer decoction which had saved so many hopeless cases was too difficult to digest. One false step might have meant death.

Finally, we decided to soak some linseed in water overnight, strain it, and give the liquid to the patient in sips, warmed to blood heat. To our relief she was able to retain this and assimilate it. We also took the risk of giving an enema, which was dangerous in her condition but essential for the cure, to reduce toxicity. Thus, we won the first round in the struggle for a human life and went on very cautiously, step by step. Potato water, whey, carrot juice, and a little mild sour milk were added, one by one, to the menu. But as soon as we tried to give the patient any solid food, we were faced by apparently insoluble problems. Then she, herself, cut the Gordian knot and asked for the flesh of overripe pears.

Providentially, we had a whole box full of overripe pears in the cellar. As long as there is a thin layer of white flesh under the skin of a pear, no putrefactive bacteria can find their way beyond it, but the inner flesh of the fruit has undergone slight fermentation, which makes it extremely easy to digest. The experiment succeeded and soon the menu could be further enriched by boiled, mashed potatoes without the skin. Potatoes, freshly boiled and warm, are one of the most easily digested foods.

When, a few weeks later, I had to leave for Germany, the patient went home. She had progressed so far that she was able to sit up for an hour or two every day. On the day of departure she had her first rusk, softened in warm milk and water.

She continued to improve for a couple of years. The old lady's daughter wrote and told us how happy her mother was in her regained health. She grew so strong that she was able to take long walks. She had no return of the disease which had overshadowed her life for so many years.

The last letter I received brought the news, however, that Mrs. M. had passed peacefully away in her sleep. Her end had been painless and easy.

Another equally severe case was that of a desperate, emaciated, hopeless invalid, Friedrich Teschemacher, who arrived at Elmau in February, 1952. He had spent most of his time in hospitals since 1941, in great suffering. This was his case history:

Severely wounded in 1941, dysentery, shrapnel in his back, sciatic nerve severed, fractured femur, severe diarrhea. He was unable to retain any food and was in the hospital for 17 months. For 4½ years he had been almost continuously in hospitals. In 1943: pus formations from the shrapnel, colon badly damaged, repeated operations, septic fevers, intestinal fistulas. He was bedridden and constantly under narcotics. In 1946, an artificial opening for the bowel was made. Periodically severe diarrhea, pain and discomfort in the stomach, disturbances of the autonomic nervous system. The patient could take no food and was extremely weak.

In this case the patient was able to take the usual decoction for gastric ulcer, which was given to him every two hours. Raw onions were chopped, wrapped in surgical gauze and placed on, or at the edges of, the suppurating shrapnel sores. The onions were renewed every three hours. Sitz baths in a camomile decoction were given every day. Instead of the carrot juice he was given a strong decoction of dried whortleberries (bilberries, or blueberries), which is very healing and astringent.

With the utmost caution we felt our way. There were many relapses, and these often meant starting again from the beginning. Planning a diet for such sick and badly damaged digestive organs is like doing a jigsaw puzzle, in that it demands infinite patience and untiring watchfulness. If the margin of what can be assimilated is overstepped, the effect is immediate. Hour by hour and day by day the patient's progress must be followed and his diet increased with the utmost care. If something he is able to digest has been found, one cannot make another advance at once but must wait until the improvement has been established. All gastric ulcers treated by this method, if they are without serious complications, should be healed after four weeks. In complicated, extremely severe cases of the nature here described, it is impossible to tell how long the healing will take.

After one month Herr Teschemacher left Elmau. He was already much better. The important thing was that we had experimented until we had found a nourishing, balanced diet on which he could build further. He was no longer so emaciated, and he had some color in his cheeks and a gleam of hope in his eye.

I saw him again after a year had passed—and did not recognize him! His face was like a rosy winter apple, his figure strong and muscular. He was a picture of health and full of vitality. We had met at the Health Week in Coblenz and when I had my famous duel with the well-known nutritionist Profesor Tropp, at the meeting in the old castle of Ehrenbreitstein, Herr Teschemacher got up and testified to how the Waerland therapy had transformed a hopeless, tortured invalid into a healthy man, full of vitality and good spirits. Herr Teschemacher is now the leader of the Waerland Movement in Germany.

Since then I have had a large number of cases in my care, not always so severe but just as slow; in fact, some of them were still more obstinate. In overcoming disease, the primary factor on which success depends is the patient's own vitality. There often are cases of illness which seem to run on a normal, apparently harmless course but which sap the patient's vitality to such an extent that to bring about a change for the better is extremely difficult.

Many cases of severe hemorrhage of the bowel have been under my care. At Bad Soden, in the autumn of 1953, we had a patient, *Herr L.*, who for many years had had severe digestive disturbances and bleeding from the bowel. We did not succeed in stopping the bleeding in the first three weeks, although it obviously came from a place low down in the rectum. The diet for ulcers brought about a general improvement although not quite the desired result. Then I tried mixing finely grated garlic with a soothing skin ointment and inserting it into the rectum as far as possible; this helped in a surprisingly short time. The patient began to improve rapidly, putting on flesh, and his strength and color returned.

At Kiholm, in the winter of 1953-1954, we had an old Norwegian lady suffering from bleeding from the bowel. The diagnosis was serious but a month's treatment worked wonders. The bleeding ceased and the old lady felt quite well.

Thus, the damage done by mistakes in living can be repaired if only the forces of nature are assisted by a diet that is at the same time cleansing, healing, and nourishing, and by internal cleansing given carefully and consistently.

Treatment of intestinal catarrh

In treating these diseases the first thing to be aimed at is to heal the mucous membranes of the intestines and strengthen their slackened muscles.

Patients suffering from intestinal catarrh have to be extremely careful as to their choice of foods. It is not possible to set up, here, a dietary that will be suitable for all cases, since each single patient must follow his own individual course, carefully testing and working out what foods can be tolerated. Then the diet must be continued until a lasting improvement has been established. A long-standing, chronic, and severe intestinal catarrh should, after about six months with our therapy, be so far healed that the patient can try the ordinary Waerland diet, with molino instead of kruska. But it is wise to live for a time on the special bland diet for patients recovering from gastric and intestinal ulcers. Always, of course, providing no complications arise which delay the healing process.

A deficiency of hydrochloric acid often accompanies intestinal catarrh, but it corrects itself spontaneously if the patient lives on a healing and nourishing bland diet. The glands of the stomach will sooner or later begin to excrete all the necessary digestive juices. A very good stimulant for these glands is raw potato juice. It should be taken, a tablespoonful at a time, shortly before meals. The remarkable thing is that, in patients with a deficiency of hydrochloric acid, it produces hydrochloric acid, and in patients who have too much, the excess hydrocloric acid is neutralized. In other words it has the capacity to restore the lost balance. Acid fruit juice, such as sour cranberry juice, cranberry jam, or a little lemon juice, can be used as substitutes for hydrochloric acid and should be taken along with the meals.

Even if the patient has diarrhea he must, for the first

month (and in some cases longer), have a daily enema, using either a camomile decoction or an addition of kaolin to the warm water. (A tablespoonful of kaolin to a pint of water.) Kaolin is a finely pulverized, whitish clay with great healing properties and has been used for centuries by the Chinese. Large-sized enemas should be taken only once or twice a week, but the small, tepid one-pint one, with a pinch of kaolin, is taken every day.

No disease demands such individual treatment as intestinal catarrh.

Diet and treatment for intestinal catarrh

For long-standing, severe catarrh the patient must fast on the gastric-ulcer decoction. It should be taken every two hours, seven times a day. If possible, a little raw carrot juice or a decoction of dried blueberries (two heaping tablespoonfuls of blueberries soaked in 2 pints of boiling water at night: in the morning boil for about twenty minutes, or until the liquid is reduced to a pint). *At lunch and dinner time* a glass of mild sour milk is given as well as the decoction.

Diet after the fast.

On waking: Half a pint (¼ liter) of the decoction with half a pint (¼ liter) of blueberry juice (prepared as described above).

Breakfast: Mild sour milk with a little carrot juice: the quantity varies according to the patient's capacity to assimilate the juice.

Midmorning & Afternoon: Decoction, or camomile tea, or rose-hip tea.

Lunch: Potatoes, boiled in jackets without salt, peeled and mashed; a little carrot juice, mild sour milk, cottage cheese; light ryvita or crisp bread, or wheat rusks; butter or a little cold-pressed oil. Possibly cooked carrots or spinach. Later on some grated raw roots.

Dinner: Boiled rice, a glass of tepid milk, wheat rusks, or light crisp bread; butter and cottage cheese.

Evening: Blueberry preparation or some soothing tea, with rusks and butter.

This diet should be gradually expanded very carefully, along the same lines as for gastric ulcer. At the evening meal, mashed potatoes may be taken as an alternative to rice.

13 / *Diseases of the liver, kidneys, and gall bladder*

If the most important organs dealing wth the elimination of waste products, the liver, kidneys, and gall bladder, have degenerated and do not function properly, we are faced with an impending catastrophe. The first essential for health is the ability to rid the body of all waste products as quickly and effectively as possible. The tiny amoeba, which has been swimming about in the oceans of the world since time began, owes its perfect health and long life to the fact that it is capable of maintaining a perfect balance between the intake of food and the elimination of waste products.

Our liver is an organ whose job it is to free the body from poisons and to neutralize all substances that could be harmful. In the body of civilized man the liver works under pressure day and night and finally succumbs through overwork. It is the same with the kidneys, which are forced to deal with an unnaturally salty and highly seasoned diet while not being supplied with sufficient fluid to dissolve and carry off the surplus. Thus poisons are formed which find their way through the blood stream to all the organs and tissues.

How can healthy sound tissues or cells be built up in a

body where waste products stagnate and accumulate and where degenerated tissues provide an ideal breeding ground for disease-causing bacteria? It is frightening to observe how greatly the diseases affecting these organs have increased in the last few years. Blindly, civilized man lays himself open not only to bodily but also to psychological ills in so far as he poisons his body and mind by habitual errors in living. The so-called delights of the palate are often obtained at the expense of health and happiness.

When the detoxicating organs have ceased to function properly, the rebuilding of health is extremely difficult and complicated. It takes a long time to restore these organs, because they are constantly being assailed by the very poisons which they should have neutralized and eliminated from the system.

The first thing to be done is to rest the organs by giving them as little work as possible. The best way of doing this is through cleansing and fasting, great care being taken to adapt and vary the treatment to suit each individual case. For, in patients who suffer from a disease affecting any one of these organs, it is usually found that other organs have been affected by the general toxicity, and these must be taken into consideration. If, for instance, the heart is affected, a rigorous fast would not be advisable. Instead, a semi-fast or light, detoxicating diet should be introduced. If the intestinal functions are disturbed and the patient is at first unable to assimilate a diet of raw vegetables and juices, which are essential for cell regeneration, it will be necessary to experiment until a suitable diet has been found containing essential food elements which the patient can assimilate.

With diseases of these organs the diet must be highly alkaline (see p. 202). Gall-bladder patients can usually take fruit, but liver patients in particular should keep to the alkaline juices of roots and green leaves. The most severe, long-standing cases of gall-bladder trouble, accompanied by vomiting, severe colic, formation of gallstones and inability to assimilate food, have often been helped by a semi-fast on the decoction of potato-and-vegetable water, ripe, unsprayed pears, and herbal teas. In less severe cases good results have been obtained with an olive-oil treatment and birch-leaf tea in conjunction with the specially adapted diet.

I should like to mention some typical cases here.

A famous Swiss artist, an elderly man of sixty-eight, arrived in a sorry condition at Sonnenhof, the Waerland sanatorium in Switzerland. He lay in bed, hollowed-eyed, emaciated and parchment-colored, unable to sleep and quite apathetic. He had lost the will to live and with it all hope, and suffered day and night from pain and torment. He had formerly painted beautiful landscapes, and the magic of his brush had opened up visions of beauty to all who saw his work. But slowly all his organs had given way through chronic poisoning. Now his body was only a tortured shell for his hopeless spirit.

For four years he had suffered from vomiting and vertigo, a typical sign of severe poisoning.

This was the natural outcome of long-standing constipation and the toxic degeneration of the liver, kidneys, and gall bladder. For several years he had also suffered from gastric ulcer. In 1951 he underwent an operation, but the abdomen was opened and closed again without removal of the diseased part. On top of all this, he had acute neuralgia and rheumatic pains. Indeed, he was suffering so much that he had given up looking for a way out of his misery and was only hoping for the end to come soon.

While I was still at Sonnenhof his treatment was started with fasting on the decoction as prescribed for gastric ulcers, stomach and intestinal diseases (see p. 198). A great deal of effort and power of persuasion were necessary before the patient could be induced to submit to the treatment and so restore his will to live, but before I left the sanatorium I was privileged to see him lying under the chestnut trees on the terrace overlooking beautiful Lake Thun. I had seen how the number of his little bottles and boxes filled with narcotics dwindled as he was helped to quiet and refreshing sleep by my simple herb tea made from salvia, hops, and camomile, which had helped so many patients before.

When I left, the proprietress of Sonnenhof, Frau Keller, took over this difficult case and achieved splendid results through her patience and devotion. She helped the patient to find his way back to life, and to the joy of creative work. I could hardly believe it when I heard that our former patient was holding another exhibition. Still another miracle had happened.

Another case was that of E.K., a man of forty, who took

refuge at Kiholm in the autumn of 1951, after having spent many years in various hospitals, being treated by the most eminent physicians. Since July, 1949, he had been suffering from Bright's disease but in spite of hospital treatment had grown steadily worse and since August, 1949, had had constant attacks of vomiting and diarrhea. His blood pressure was high, as were also his blood sedimentation and soluble-nitrogen rate. He was treated with injections of aminosol and was given Hydrogan, after which his whole body became swollen. Then he sought the advice of two well-known professors at Uppsala, under whose treatment he lived for a time on a diet consisting entirely of butter, sugar, and a little water (200 grams of butter and 200 grams of sugar daily). In January, 1950, he went into the Academic Hospital at Uppsala, where he was given makrodex (a solution of sugar). During the eighteen months of his illness he had had sixty blood transfusions, with the addition of makrodex and aminosol. During the whole time he spent in the hospital he had continuous vomiting. He was eventually moved from Uppsala to the hospital at Eskilstuna in May, 1950, where he lay until the middle of July. In the spring of 1950 his blood sedimentation rate was 157, the Esbach test for quantitative albumin 24, serum albumin 2.4. In November, 1950, the blood sedimentation was 116, serum protein 5.3 non-protein nitrogen 71, and blood pressure 180.

The patient was admitted to Kiholm on November 26, 1950. By December 10 the Esbach test had fallen to 9.

Unfortunately, he was unable to stay longer than three weeks, but even in that time his condition was marvelously improved through fasting, bowel cleansing and, afterward, a diet very low in protein but highly alkaline and rich in vitamins and minerals. When he left Kiholm, the blood sedimentation rate was 100, blood pressure 142, serum albumin 4.9, non-protein nitrogen 38 and, what was most astonishing, the hemoglobin count was 90%.

Frau V., age sixty, was from Garmisch-Partenkirchen. She had leukemia, myocarditis, and disturbances of the liver. In 1951 she had had a nervous breakdown with paralytic symptoms. This was treated with injections which caused painful cramp in the capillaries. Besides this she had unrelieved insomnia. By changing over to the Waerland diet she got much better and when, later on, she went to Elmau and was given my cure for liver patients, she completely recovered. The action of the heart was assisted by the administration of tincture of Crataegus, a homeopathic remedy which built up the heart muscle. The normal blood count was restored by the high content of chlorophyll and minerals in the diet. These results were backed up by supplementary vitamin B_{12} and sleep was induced by the hop-salvia-camomile tea. The patient was soon able to go on to the normal Waerland diet glowing with vitality and became a living proof of the soundness of our principles.

In conclusion I should like to describe a case which clearly shows that the kidney disturbances leading to a secretion of albumen can be cured by a rightly composed diet but also that a relapse will immediately follow as soon as undue strain is put on the kidneys by a return to wrong foods.

A few years ago, at the beginning of May, a young German woman, Frau Ackerman, came to consult me. She and her husband had come to Sweden as refugees. The husband was employed at Uppsala and had been cured of various ailments by the Waerland diet after years of bad health. His young wife, however, had not adopted the new diet with her husband, which eventually cost her dear. In the second month of her pregnancy she showed signs of albuminuria which grew steadily worse. She was under the observation of the Academic Hospital at Uppsala. In the fifth month of her pregnancy the albumen content was so high that she had to be admitted to the hospital where, after three weeks, she had a miscarriage. The hospital authorities explained to her that she must on no account attempt another pregnancy, as she belonged to the dangerous Rh. negative blood group. Women belonging to this group seldom bear children fit to survive and when they do it depends on the blood group of the marriage partner. Even if the pregnancy is completed the child is in many cases stillborn and, if not, the chief possibility of saving the child is for a complete change of blood to be made immediately after the birth. There is only one hospital in Sweden, the Karolinska hospital in Stockholm, where this kind of transfusion can be carried out. This drastic step is the only means orthodox medicine has yet found to help unhappy mothers of this group.

It was not long, however, before Frau Ackerman was

pregnant again. In the third month, as before, the high content of albumen appeared, and in the sixth month the doctors again insisted on her entering the hospital. She knew what she would have to face there and in desperation turned to me for advice. Until then I had never even heard of these complicated cases and I told her that I did not think I could help her. The only thing, in my opinion, that might help her would be to relieve the strain on the kidneys. The excessive albumen was, after all, only the outward sign of the serious functional disturbance in these organs. In view of this, I suggested my special diet for kidney ailments which had been giving excellent results for several years.

Some doctors are of the opinion that in these cases the patient should be given a diet containing plenty of protein to make up for the continual loss of it in the urine. My own opinion is that the opposite is applicable. The diet should be as low in protein content as possible for patients with Bright's disease, for whom I reduce the daily ration of milk to under one pint. The rest of the diet consists of mild alkaline foods, with as much green salad as the patient can assimilate, and plenty of root vegetable juices and, when available, diluted nettle and dandelion juice. These patients usually have a mild raw meal both at midday and for supper.

I advised Frau Ackerman not to wait too long but to visit the hospital quite soon again for a check-up. On her way back to Uppsala, sitting in the train by an open window, she was suddenly startled by another train passing in the opposite direction and—felt her water break. In despair she rang me up from Uppsala. I begged her to return to Stockholm at once and then met her and took her by car to the Karolinska hospital. But, because she had not been sent by a doctor, no one would have anything to do with her and she was finally sent back to the Academic Hospital in Uppsala. The baby would be "beyond help" anyway, she was told.

However, as the birth did not seem to be imminent, Frau Ackerman waited a few days before she went to the hospital, strictly adhering to my diet meanwhile. At the hospital she was greeted with reproaches for not coming sooner but, on examining her, they were astonished to find that the protein content had not risen. A further examination a few days later even showed a slight improvement, and after a couple of weeks the albumen had disappeared entirely, to the amazement of the doctors and nurses.

This happened at the beginning of June. At the end of August, Frau Ackerman gave birth to a healthy, normal child. Her confinement at the Academic Hospital was normal and the delivery was unusually quick and easy. I believe that her case, which was unique of its kind, aroused a good deal of interest among the doctors and nurses. They were obliging enough to promise her a raw-vegetable diet—but what did that mean? Consisting mainly of large quantities of milk and grapefruit, it was most unsuitable for her weakened, easily irritated, and overworked kidneys, and the consequences were not long in coming. After only a few days' stay at the hospital, not only did the albuminuria reappear but she became constipated as well, from which trouble she had been quite free before her confinement, thanks to a correct diet.

This condition persisted as long as she stayed at the hospital, but as soon as she had settled down at home, with her bowel rhythm restored, and was back on her special kidney diet, the albumen disappeared. The baby was splendid and continued to develop normally.

Doctors are completely baffled by these difficult cases of Bright's disease in pregnant women of the Rh. negative blood group and have found no natural way of saving the babies. Yet, when I went to see the head of our famous Maternity Hospital in Stockholm and asked that my methods be tried out there under his supervision, he refused.

What, then, are the principles on which our treatment is based—a treatment which so effectively cures and regenerates our great detoxicating organs? They are so simple that everyone should be able to grasp them:

1. We try in every way to assist the body's own cleansing processes.
2. We give a diet which is protective and nonirritating to the diseased organ and at the same time builds it up. Kidney patients should, above all, reduce protein consumption while liver and gall affections call for a reduction of fats. Salt and all acid or acid-forming foods must be avoided. The diet must contain an abundance of nutritious elements such as vitamins, minerals, chlorophyll, trace, elements and auxones, besides which it should be highly alkaline.

The most important feature of the treatment is the assistance given to the broken-down detoxicating organs by means of enemas and properly administered colonic irrigation. It is essential to rest the diseased organs and the digestive tract so that all the regenerative forces of the body may be devoted to the cure.

We must see to it that the patients have not only an adequate diet but fresh, pure air free from poisonous fumes and tobacco smoke, and water that is not polluted by drains or so-called disinfectants. An ailing liver cannot possibly neutralize all the poisons which civilized people habitually introduce into the body by every means of ingress.

Treatment and diet for gall, liver, and kidney diseases

In treating all these diseases, enemas and colonic irrigation are indispensable and should be given systematically until a steady improvement is noticeable. At the beginning of the treatment the patient should have an enema night and morning, first a small quantity of about a pint, which is expelled at once, and then the enema proper, about two pints. In cases of gall-bladder and liver trouble the patients must be extremely careful with all kinds of fat, and kidney patients with proteins.

Gall-bladder diseases

The most effective means is a fast (according to instructions in Chapter 23).

Severe cases of long standing respond best to a treatment consisting of ripe, unsprayed pears. For from three to eight days, the patient takes no solid food except pears. These are eaten at mealtimes. The patient may eat as many pears as he tolerates. In between, he drinks about two quarts of liquid daily, consisting of potato water, horsetail tea, and tea made from nettles or dandelions. Enema morning and evening during the pear treatment (longer if necessary). After the prescribed number of days the patient is put on a highly alkaline diet rich in chlorophyll but low in fats. This diet should be as follows:

On waking: Drink "*Excelsior*" (p. 199).

Breakfast: Sour milk with wheat bran; powdered nettles or rose hips, milk sugar. Carrot juice or sweet fruit (acid fruit should be avoided).

Midmorning & Midafternoon: Tea—from horsetail, dandelion, or nettles.

Lunch: Rawkost (but no onions or leeks, nor any root vegetable with strong flavor, such as horse-radish), potatoes, and a glass of sour milk. Raw juices of carrots, dandelion, and nettles; bread as for rheumatics, or crisp bread. No ordinary cheese or butter but a little cold-pressed oil and some cottage cheese (recipe p. 197).

Dinner: The same menu as for lunch or, for a change, potato porridge (recipe p. 205) with a little mild stewed fruit and a glass of milk. Alternatively, if desired, rice kruska or molino.

Gall-bladder patients should note that it is absolutely

essential for them to have bowel movements two or three times a day.

Liver diseases

The diet for these patients is similar to that for gall-bladder patients, but still greater care must be taken with regard to fats, and therefore even the cold-pressed oil must be avoided at first.

Kidney diseases

These patients also have a similar diet, but in their case it is essential to reduce protein foods, i.e., milk and cheese. At most they should drink a pint of milk per day. No cheese whatever is allowed.

14 / Multiple sclerosis

This disease is undoubtedly one of the worst of the "diseases of civilization." It is a nerve disease arising through injuries to the white substances of the brain and of the spinal marrow. These injuries are, to a large extent, the result of unnatural, unbalanced diet which poisons the organism on the one hand and is lacking in vital substances on the other. The fact that so many young people develop the disease may be partially due to inherited weaknesses from parents whose organisms are deficient in vital body-building elements. And the fact that other nervous diseases have also become so prevalent among civilized races is no doubt attributable to the same causes, aggravated by the effects of world-shattering wars and the stress of modern life. No more poignant evidence of the need for education in right living can be found than these terrible diseases.

The first doctor to recognize the importance of diet in treating multiple sclerosis was Dr. Evers, in Germany. He was able to arrest the course of the disease and in many cases gradually succeeded in building up new health in the patient. He advocates abstention from all foods which have passed through manufacturing processes and recommends raw vegetables in the diet. Thus far his method follows the same principles as our own. Dr. Evers, however, gives his patients raw meat and raw egg yolk, while forbidding potatoes and green salads. The potatoes and salads are most important constituents of a full, all-round, health-building diet, while raw meat and yolk of egg introduce putrefactive bacteria into the organism. This is probably why Dr. Evers' otherwise effective diet has not had even better results.

The only effective way of arresting the course of the disease and restoring the patient to health is to rid the body of poisons and supply it with the elements of regeneration. In addition it is important to stimulate the circulation, digestive processes, and metabolism by therapeutic exercises, massage, and baths. The patient himself can contribute enormously to his recovery. Step by step he must fight on with unceasing energy to revivify his numbed muscles. Infinite endurance and patience are called for, and easily gained, rapid results must not be expected.

It was in the Bavarian Alps, at the sanatorium of Elmau, that I first met I.G., a young girl, in the spring of 1951. This sanatorium was then being run by Dr. E. Röhling, a German doctor who had spent a couple of months at Kiholm, our Swedish sanatorium, to study our diet treatment. In an advanced stage of multiple sclerosis, I.G. was a pitiable sight, broken down in mind and body and completely without hope. When one tried to encourage her, floods of tears were her only reply.

She was in Dr. Röhling's care for that summer and was already much improved when I took over on the first of

October. Before long she was able to help us in the house and by the end of November was in such good form that she was able to set out alone on a mountain climb in snow and ice. She started off at dawn and did not return until late in the evening after an achievement that would be envied by many a person in good health.

A young Swiss woman came to the Sonnenhof Sanatorium at Thun, having had multiple sclerosis for many years. Thanks to the Waerland diet she recovered sufficiently to live a normal life and is now settled in Sweden with her Swedish husband.

Another patient at the Sonnenhof, the forty-year-old Frau A.B., made a remarkable recovery in only three weeks, but it must be added that she had only been ill for one year.

My first patient in Germany was Herr Fritz Rösch. He was suffering not from multiple sclerosis but from a paralytic disease with many similar features in its nature and development. The course of his illness gives us an explanation of the cause and development of these paralytic diseases.

For eight years Herr Rösch had been in a hospital with constantly increasing paralysis which gradually spread all over his body. During the second world war he had had a series of inoculations against various diseases, and these had broken down his health. The paralysis began in his legs and slowly spread until the intestines and bladder were almost paralyzed. This was the worst thing that could have happened, as it put two of the most important functions of elimination out of action, so that almost all residues and accumulated poisons were retained in the body.

At the hospital nothing had been done to empty the bowel daily, and the intervals between evacuations became longer, the bowel more distended and relaxed. The patient was unable to pass water and a catheter had to be used. He dreaded this so much that he drank as little as possible. This was successful in so far as the painful procedure was less frequently required; but on the other hand his bladder, highly important in the process of elimination, became a focal point of infection. The disease now had full play in his body. The paralysis crept on to his arms, one of which became completely paralyzed and the other shook so that he could not use it. But this was not enough: the paralysis spread to the brain, so that he was unable to speak coherently and stammered.

In this condition Herr Rösch came to Dietz an der Lahn, where I was staying on my first visit to Germany after the war. I had been invited to the Felkes Sanatorium in Dietz to introduce the Waerland diet. There were no bedrooms in the main building, but the patients slept in outdoor huts which were, however, so dilapidated that the rain came in through roof and walls. The dining rooms were in the main building, which was otherwise full of troops of the occupation armies. It was a ten-minute walk from the huts. There was no nursing staff and no resident doctor.

Herr Rösch came from a hospital in Berne, having traveled in an ambluance compartment on the train and by motor ambulance from the station at Dietz. He was then carried on a stretcher to one of the huts.

It all looked hopeless. But there was nothing for it but to grit one's teeth and try to help the poor sufferer until he could be taken home again.

First I wanted to do all I could to restore his organs of elimination to natural functioning. This, I could see, was the only possibility of saving his life. I undertook the nursing myself. In spite of the great risk there was no other alternative than to begin with a fast on alkaline raw juices and vegetable broths, while trying to clear the reservoirs of poisons in the bladder and bowels. This might have seemed impossible, since both were paralyzed. The bowel was unable to retain the enema fluid, which ran out as fast as it went in. Only after endless effort and many failures a little water was finally induced to enter the atrophied bowel and soften the stagnant excrement. By degrees larger quantities of water were retained and the cleansing of the intestinal tract was begun.

The greatest stumbling block was, however, the bladder. It had not functioned naturally for years and was unable to cope with the unaccustomed fluid intake, which stagnated, with accompanying cramp. A doctor had to be called in to empty the bladder artificially. We had brought on a dangerous crisis but it was only through this crisis that the road to health lay. The bladder had to be forced to resume its function. Naturally we had to begin with very small rations of fluid but were soon able to increase them. Our bold attempt succeeded: the bladder began to empty itself spontaneously. At first a thick, dark, evil-smelling fluid was expelled, but the urine soon became clearer, lighter in color, and more profuse.

The battle was now won—the first round at all events. The two most important organs had resumed work. Results were not long in coming. After a short time the paralyzed arm began to show signs of life and the other arm did not shake so much. The patient was able to sit up in bed and hold a glass or cup. Hanging by the arms on the shoulders of two people, he could be got across the room.

He was under my care for only ten days before he journeyed by ambulance and train back to Switzerland, but even in that short time a radical change had taken place. He was no longer a man marked out by death. He had entered the path that was to lead him out of the inferno of suffering. The regenerating forces of his own body had taken the upper hand.

Is it not true that so-called "civilized people" do all they can to hinder these forces and give the forces of destruction free play?

Herr Rösch went to stay with a family in Berne who looked after him in accordance with my instructions. Two years later I visited him. He was radiant with gratitude as he told me about his daily walks, his peaceful life, his interests and recreations. He was now enjoying such health as he could not have dreamed possible during those long years in the hospital.

The cases of multiple sclerosis that we have seen respond to this type of treatment are too numerous to describe in detail here, but there is one more recent case, still talked of at Kiholm—that of Harry Berglund. From the first indications in 1940 until the autumn of 1954, when he he came to us, he had been in and out of hospitals and undergone all the most modern treatments. Multiple sclerosis is intermittent in its manner of development, advancing in waves and leaving the patient a little worse after each wave. Berglund's case was no exception to this, and in addition he had had heart weakness, goitre, jaundice, and pneumonia. Before coming to Kiholm, he had been trying the Waerland methods himself but found that diet alone was not sufficient and he must have expert guidance. He was with us for two months and his treatment started with five days' fasting with raw juices—the longest period we allow for multiple-sclerosis patients. He began to improve during the fast and afterward had two rawkost meals a day plus sprouted wheat grains. In three to four weeks he abandoned his cane. Other features of his treatment were enemas and colonic irrigation (ten of the latter during the two-month stay), also daily exercises and massage. He entered into the treatment with understanding and persevered with his own physical training, timing his walks and gradually increasing their length while shortening the time. During his stay with us he improved steadily and was better than he had been for many years when the time came for him to return home. No break was made in the daily routine, and the improvement continued. The stiff climb from the bridge over the river up to the farmyard, a distance of eight hundred meters (about a half mile), he made in a half hour when he came home from Kiholm, but he soon did it in twenty minutes. He now faces the future with calm assurance, aware of the incredible change that has taken place in his body, not merely the easing of pain and freedom of movement, but a new sense of well-being and alertness, and he no longer wavers between hope and fear.

From one of our doctors in Germany I learned of the case of Frau F., who had a paralytic disease known scientifically as *Myasthenia gravis pseudoparalytica* and considered incurable. Its victims usually die of pneumonia when the paralysis reaches the breathing muscles. This being a very rare disease and consequently of particular interest, Frau F. was offered a free bed in the university clinic in Hamburg.

The patient soon felt that she could not expect any improvement there, but at that time came in contact with Waerland ideas through some pamphlets she read. These opened up a new perspective and she took courage. In spite of protests from the doctors, she left the hospital and began to treat herself according to directions in our literature. In the course of a year she fasted, in various short periods, altogether thirteen weeks. Each period of fasting brought an improvement in her condition, and after eighteen months the disease had almost left her, only reminding her now and then, if she overexerted herself, by a slight paralysis of one side of her face.

Modifications of diet for cases of multiple sclerosis and other paralytic diseases

After a short fast, which may be repeated at intervals, the patients must have an exclusively alkaline diet, i.e., two rawkost meals daily with the addition of sprouted wheat grains (for preparation see p. 208).

Later, for a change, the ordinary Waerland diet* may be taken for a week or two with added sprouted wheat grains.

For these patients, bread must be reduced to one or two slices daily. Only bread baked with sourdough is permitted. Cold-pressed oil should preferably be used instead of butter. No cheese except homemade cottage or whey cheese (see p. 197). Sugar should be avoided, but honey is allowed in very small quantities.

If unpasteurized milk is unobtainable, it is better to keep to two rawkost meals.

These patients must take particular care to avoid all refined and denatured foods. They should have plentiful doses of vitamin B. This is extremely important. Brewer's yeast is recommended.

* See Chap. 3.

15 / Dropsy

Dropsy is the result of advanced degeneration in the body, the metabolic turnover of fluids having been disorganized through the weakening of certain vital organs, which are no longer able to carry out their function. The stagnation of unhealthy fluids in the tissues is often due to weakness of the heart, when the blood stream is not driven with sufficient force through the arteries and veins, and the cells are not supplied with the necessary quantities of oxygen and nourishment. This results in general stagnation, with catastrophic consequences. In most cases the liver and kidneys also refuse to function properly. In their overstrained condition they are unable to excrete the accumulating waste products of metabolism. Hence, dropsy is a typical impurity disease, arising from overloading and poisoning of our most important organs: heart, liver, and kidneys. It can be cured only by going to the root of the evil and trying to detoxicate the body by means of suitable fasting and cleansing processes. These must, however, be undertaken with the utmost care and individual attention, since fasting is fraught with certain risks in cases where there is weakness of the heart muscles. It is therefore advisable to support the functioning of the heart by a homeopathic remedy such as, for instance, crataegus mother tincture. Crataegus is produced from hawthorn and has been used in the art of healing since ancient times. Well-known authorities consider that crataegus will give better results even than digitalis. Used in conjunction with a wholesome, detoxicating diet, it will work wonders.

Naturally a patient suffering from dropsy is not able to take such large quantities of fluids as we otherwise recommend. A heart and kidneys on strike can tolerate only very small and slowly consumed drinks, but, as the elimination of poisons proceeds, these organs must be trained to deal with increased quantities of liquid. The excretory organs cannot fulfill their task without plenty of fluids.

In advanced cases of dropsy it is usually necessary for the patient to undergo a puncture in order to relieve the body of the unhealthy fluids collected in the tissues. These fluids not only put a great strain on the degenerated organs but also are bad for the whole organism. An immediate improvement can be noticed after the puncture has removed the strain from the seat of the poisoning, but this relief does not usually last long, in which case the puncture will have to be repeated after a few days. A whole series of punctures often brings no improvement under the ordinary, orthodox treatment of dropsy; but this is due to the fact that the diet given does not support the detoxicating processes, often even hampering the healing forces of the body. If, on the other hand, these forces are assisted by effective cleansing and a fast on alkaline juices rich in vitamins and minerals, it will be found that, even in the most advanced cases, only two or three punctures are usually necessary.

After the fast has been broken, the patient's diet must be adapted entirely to his condition and his ability to assimilate foods. No general rules can, therefore, be given. It usually means taking special care on account of impaired kidneys and liver and weakened digestive organs.

My first dropsy patient was Mrs. A. K. She had already gone through decades of suffering before I met her. At the age of eighteen she had contracted severe arthritis. Gradually, the overworked liver became inflamed and the heart became seriously affected, with muscular weakness and enlargement. At various times the patient had been treated in hospitals, but it had not been possible to arrest the development of the disease, which had steadily worsened until it had culminated in dropsy. When the patient arrived at Kiholm, her condition was extremely critical owing to the state of her heart. Fortunately she had a friend with her who watched over her night and day.

Two tapping operations drew off altogether about eleven quarts of fluid from her body. The first of these was done at the hospital in Södertälje, where the officiating doctor had no faith in, or understanding of, natural healing. He refused to let her return to Kiholm.

But the patient had been treated for a very long time at the hospital in her home town, where it was proposed to send her, and all the usual methods had been tried in vain, so she had no desire to go back. All her hopes were fixed on Kiholm and our treatment. How she and her friend, two elderly ladies, succeeded in breaking down the opposition of the doctor I never knew, but, to my amazement, they returned to Kiholm a few days after my telephone conversation with the doctor.

The second tapping operation was done at Kiholm by Dr. Östling, the physician who has made it possible for us to receive and successfully treat so many desperate, abandoned cases.

Mrs. A. K. was unable to fast, her heart being too seriously affected. Instead, she was put on a semi-fast (the result of several years' experimenting on my part) now known to us as the *limited diet* (see instructions on p. 201).

During this semi-fast the patient has no solid food before noon. *The morning drink* consists of an alkaline decoction of vegetables and potatoes, sometimes with linseed and bran added. To begin with, only small amounts can be taken at a time, about half a pint, slowly increasing up to a pint if the heart allows. The patient should always drink very slowly.

Breakfast: Should consist solely of fruit—unsprayed, of course—e.g., apples, oranges, or berries, with a cup of herb tea or, alternatively, raw carrot juice or other vegetable juice instead of the fruit and tea. Carrot juice is usually the easiest for the patient to tolerate.

Lunch and Dinner: Rawkost—as much as can be managed by the patient, a few small potatoes, a glass of sour milk, a little raw juice, a little cottage cheese but no butter, no ordinary cheese and very little bread—only a slice of wholemeal bread at dinner.

This extremely light, alkaline diet brings about a process

of cleansing which to a certain extent takes the place of a regular fast. Enemas should be given morning and evening during the first weeks. Afterward, a small, cool enema of one pint is given in the evening only (within half an hour after the evening meal). It is important that the water should be cool—but not too cold—as this promotes a certain stimulation of the nerves of the rectum which in its turn brings about a contraction of the muscles of the intestine, resulting in an evacuation. The best time for this is after a meal when peristalsis is active and the contents of the bowels are being carried toward the exit.

With the aid of this semi-fast and the internal cleansing, while at the same time the heart was being supported by the crataegus tincture, the healing forces of nature were given free play in Mrs. A. K. Improvement came surprisingly soon, bringing the return of sleep, a calmer heart, appetite, and better functioning of intestine and bladder. At last the patient was able to sit up. Her eyes were bright and there was color in her cheeks.

After only a month she was able to return to her family and had recovered sufficiently to take over the housekeeping. This was one of the greatest miracles I have seen.

Mrs. T. S., born 1890, had very severe dropsy. She came to Sonnenhof in 1953 after almost thirty years of suffering. As far back as 1926 she had had valvular trouble, followed by enlargement of the heart and difficulty in breathing. Then followed enlargement of the liver, and reduced liver functioning, and weakness of the bladder. As a result of all these disturbances in the body, dropsy developed. In spite of treatments in various spas and sanatoria, her condition grew worse. When Mrs. S. came to us she was like a skeleton, but her abdomen was enormously distended and as hard as a drum.

Our doctor advised against a puncture, as he considered the patient too weak and did not think the heart would stand the strain. But, because he regarded the case as hopeless, he gave in to my entreaties and made the puncture. The result was splendid. At the first puncture the patient was tapped of eleven liters (about 11½ quarts) and at the second, a few days later, a further eight and a half quarts was drawn off. Mrs. S. had undergone tapping many times before, without any resulting benefit, and now she submitted to the measure with great reluctance and little hope.

Contrary to her expectations a complete change in her condition took place. The bladder began to function spontaneously. Appetite and sleep returned. The intestine was being cleansed by means of enemas and the resistance of the body strengthened by a light, antitoxic diet. The whole organism was enabled to carry out the work of drainage through the renewed functioning of bladder and bowel, together with the easing of the strain on the kidneys by the diet. No further puncture was needed.

As she grew stronger and her condition improved, the patient became more confident. At last she had found the way that led to health, away from the suffering that had held her bound for so long. She left us firmly determined to carry out the instructions she had received and to establish her health more firmly. Later we heard that she did so.

16 / *Tuberculosis of the lungs*

Tuberculosis of the lungs is a much more widespread disease than most people realize. Most of us have, in fact, at some time had the beginnings of T.B. in such a mild form that it was not noticed.

The elderly have as a rule reached a certain immunity to the disease and are not so easily infected as young people and children. The danger of infection is especially great for babies, as they have not yet developed natural immunity. The same often applies to young people who are apparently in excellent health.

In order to eliminate the risk of infection, the Calmette vaccination has been introduced in many countries. This measure is just as unnatural and hazardous to health as vaccination for smallpox. Statistics from the various countries tell their own story about the results. A risk is taken whenever such poisons are introduced into the pure body of a baby; injections of this kind lower the resistance and prepare the soil for the so-called diseases of civilization.

In most other diseases it is necessary to counteract the abnormal acidity of the organism by a highly alkaline diet. But in treating tuberculosis of the lungs it is best to give the ordinary Waerland diet,* with kruska and plenty of

* See "Daily Program for Health," Chap. 3.

bread. For, in this case, the patient needs an acid-forming diet. After having arrived at this conclusion myself, by way of experiment and reasoning, I was delighted to hear that orthodox medicine had come to a similar conclusion. Good results are obtained by allowing the patients to inhale the fumes of acids, and it is said that employees in factories where acids are used never contract T.B. Those who already have the disease soon recover and there are never any relapses.

A bowl of wine vinegar kept standing under the patient's bed is what we advise, the fumes of vinegar being very beneficial. The vinegar must be replaced as soon as it evaporates.

Calcium is an important item in treating lung tuberculosis on account of its value in healing the cavities. Synthetic calcium preparations cannot, however, be utilized by the organism, which can only assimilate calcium in organic form. There is an old fashioned recipe which fills this want:

> Place two eggs in a china bowl with the juice of four lemons. Then put the bowl in a cool place and cover with a plate. Turn the eggs every other day. After six days the lemon juice will have drawn the calcium out of the eggs and they can be thrown away. The patient takes two tablespoonfuls of the juice every day. Every third day two more eggs are laid in lemon juice and thus the treatment can be continued for several weeks at a time.

Lung patients need a plentiful and nourishing diet. *They cannot fast.* The ordinary Waerland diet with kruska and wholemeal bread, plenty of rawkost—in which *sauerkraut* (recipe on p. 206) should not be lacking—plenty of milk and milk products, and fruit, is ideal. Onions are particularly valuable on account of their disinfecting properties. If the patient is able to tolerate garlic, he should eat some every day, trying to see how much he can take.

Of all herbs, tea made from horsetail is best for lung patients. It contains silicon, which is healing and very beneficial where blood is being coughed up. This tea is also useful when there is fever.

Even a consumptive needs to get some exercise in the fresh air if he is able. He must not, of course, overexert himself but should train himself cautiously to get up and take short walks as soon as he feels strong enough to make the effort. It is a mistake to lie in bed all the time. Gradually the walks should be extended. What a consumptive needs more than anything else is fresh air day and night. Both in summer and winter the windows should be wide open, and in warm weather he should sleep out of doors.

It is unfortunate that, in general, none of the lung sanatoria have yet introduced a reformed diet as part of the treatment of tuberculosis. In most of them it is impossible for patients to have natural, biologic food and, at the time of writing this, we have, regrettably, no special Waerland sanatorium for this disease. Those who wish to adopt our methods must treat themselves at home. In spite of this, many people with T.B. have cured themselves by our methods. Here, briefly, is a well-known case:

Nisse Öst, the well-known sportsman and tracker, late

one autumn caught a very severe cold during one of his training runs. This turned to pleurisy and he was laid up for almost a year. His general condition deteriorated all the time, and finally an examination revealed open tuberculosis of the lungs, with large cavities. Both lungs were affected, and the doctor ordered him to be sent at once to a sanatorium, but Nisse Öst had heard of the Waerland system and understood that a change-over to this diet would be his only salvation. He resolutely decided to take his fate into his own hands. He was living in a suburb of Stockholm where the air was pure and bracing, and where he could have the peace he needed in order to build up his health.

He now began eagerly to study the Waerland literature and carefully followed the directions. He cleared away all the residues and toxins by drinking copiously, including raw juices, and by means of enemas. Plenty of rest and sleep alternated with exercise in the fresh air.

It was not long before he realized that he was on the right road. The fever went and his strength began to return. After only a year he was able to begin working again.

Six months later he went on a long, strenuous skiing trip with a friend in Northern Sweden. They covered three hundred kilometers (close to two hundred miles) of rough terrain, but he stood the test splendidly in spite of severe hardships, which might have been too much for even a robust person.

Repeated X-ray examinations have shown that his lungs are now completely healed. He had himself examined regularly for several years. The doctors and nursing staff were amazed that by such simple means he had been able to cure himself of the already far-advanced disease. It was no less surprising that he remained well and had no relapse in spite of all the grueling tests to which he put himself.

A year or so after he had recovered, he entered a competition for the championship in night tracking. He had to cover a distance of five kilometers at top speed while carrying a large rucksack. And he won the first prize.

One of our first adherents in Switzerland, later on a leading member of our movement there, cured himself of a very old, long-standing tuberculosis of the lungs by our methods. Many similar instances could be given. Only a short while ago I received a letter from Germany in which Frau M. describes how she cured herself of T.B., which had been flaring up every now and then for ten years. She was undergoing treatment in a sanatorium when a relapse was confirmed. In spite of the protests of her doctors and fellow patients, she decided, as Nisse Öst had done, to take her destiny into her own hands. With great energy and patience she carried out our diet principles and our methods of treatment. The result was excellent. Two well-known specialists confirmed that she was completely well, both of them spontaneously expressing the same opinion: "If one did not know from the X-ray that there had been a cavity in the lung, one would have denied that it could have existed."

"Truly, this is a miracle," the letter goes on. "I am no longer young, already forty. Now I am quite convinced that it is possible to cure *all* diseases by means of a natural way of living and a diet along your principles, and that, in this way, a new life can be given to suffering human beings."

No one could have written in this way without having experienced the rebirth which a natural, biologic diet and a healthy way of living brings with it. All those who are still the slaves of unhealthy habits of eating and living will not be able to understand her. For them, the way to health and true joy in living is still barred. Would that this book might be so convincing as a witness to the importance of our daily habits with regard to food and the arrangement of our lives that the eyes of its readers might be opened and they, themselves, be seized with the longing to experience a new lease of life! For indeed, it is a new life, a deliverance from pain and death that many despairing people find when they reshape their lives. Let me tell of yet another case:

Herr St., a German soldier, born in 1916, fell ill with peritonitis in 1939. As a consequence of this he contracted tuberculosis of the peritoneum. This spread all through the body until almost all the organs were affected, the glandular system, the digestive tract, the kidneys, and the bladder. He had to undergo many operations and often hovered between life and death. On seven different occasions his parents were urgently summoned to his bedside. Finally he returned to his home a complete invalid. His life was a misery to himself and all about him. One kidney had been removed and the other was affected. The urinary bladder was so shriveled that it could not hold more than a few drops of fluid and emptied itself every two or three minutes.

Herr St. then heard of the Waerland system from his brother, who had also been very ill and had cured himself by a change of diet. As a drowning man, he clutched at this straw. It meant a hard struggle and passing through severe crises after the change of diet, but he stuck to his guns and finally the reward came. He is now a new man, able to be up and even occupy himself with some light work.

The most remakable feature of his case is that the ureter has built up a new bladder underneath the old one. And this new bladder can open and close. This is a fact which has been confirmed by several doctors. The new bladder functions normally and is able to hold the urine for several hours. Surely no one could hope to experience a greater miracle than this!

Colds and other respiratory diseases should have some mention here.

The mucous membrane is one of the most important excretory organs. When the body has been subjected to such sudden or severe chill that its functioning has slowed down or become stagnant, it tries to rid itself of accumulated waste matter by increasing the excretion of mucus. A cold in the head, or bronchitis, follows, perhaps with fever. What is fever except the burning up of waste matter? A radical cleansing action! Fever now is often artificially induced and brings about a surprisingly swift improvement by burning up the disease-producing toxins. I know a young man who had rheumatoid arthritis which only grew worse in spite of repeated and long spells in hospitals and various treatments and medications. Only when a delayed childish complaint brought on a high fever did the arthritis depart as if by magic and he became quite well. Artificially induced fever has the same effect.

Obviously, in view of what has just been said, nothing is more unnatural than to try to reduce fever by means of poisonous drugs in the form of powders and medicaments. Instead, every effort should be made to assist the action of the fever. This is best done by relieving the body of the effort of digestion. The only foods that should be taken are raw juices and sour milk, which have a detoxicating action and supply the body with vitamins and minerals. Fruit juices may also be given when there is fever but never at the same time as the vegetable juices. The bowel must be cleansed by enemas, and in cases of angina, inflammation of the throat, or constriction due to quinzy, etc., a light herbal laxative may even be used to aid the enemas. Perspiration and wet packs are very beneficial. In case of local inflammations the cabbage poultice or compress is invaluable. (See p. 196.)

Here, as with all other diseases, it is a matter of backing up the healing forces of nature and not loading the organism with poisonous "foreign" substances in the form of medicaments. Even the synthetic vitamin preparations are apt to disturb the balance of the body by their strong concentration and one-sidedness. Nowhere but in nature can vitamins be obtained in a properly balanced form.

Nature must be our teacher and we must bow before her infinitely wise laws. If we follow them we shall have the privilege of experiencing the complete, undreamed-of health which is our lost inheritance.

17 / *Headache, migraine, insomnia, and constipation*

These troubles are due to accumulated impurities and usually yield to treatment with balanced diet and cleansing.

Migraine and headache

As I have stated in my own case history, I suffered from continual attacks of migraine for a large part of my life. For the first three days I would have excruciating pain in the head, neck, shoulders and back, caused by cramp in the capillaries, accompanied by nausea. At the beginning of an attack the vision is distorted and one sees only half of everything. This is followed by a mist over the eyes, pierced by "lightning" flashes.

It takes time to cure such severe migraine completely, but after the change of diet the attacks become shorter and the intervals longer until they cease altogether. In very obstinate cases it may take up to a couple of years to effect a cure.

The quickest way to rid the body of the toxins which, circulating in the blood stream, cause the cramp in the capillaries, is a fast on alkaline raw juices plus internal cleansing by means of enemas or irrigation. This treatment is very swift in action, often curing a chronic headache in five to seven days. It may take longer if the short cut of the fast is not taken, and the time varies, naturally, with individual patients.

An additional means of relieving acute pain in the head is a compress made of cabbage leaves. The savoy cabbage is best, but if it is not available, ordinary white cabbage will do. The large veins are removed from the leaves, which are then crushed with a rolling pin or a bottle and laid flat on the head with edges overlapping; the leaves are then covered with a handkerchief and, over that, a piece of cotton wool or woolen stuff is placed and the whole secured with a bandage. The leaves should be renewed when withered.

Hot foot baths and alternately hot-and-cold bathing of feet and arms are also effective in drawing the blood from the head. The contrast between the hot and cold water should be as great as possible. The feet and lower part of the legs, or the arms up to the elbows, should be held for one minute in hot water and then half a minute in cold.

If the patient is able to stand steam baths, they will be found helpful in stimulating the circulation and eliminating poisons.

Typical cases

Mrs. A. H., a Finnish lady aged forty, who had suffered since childhood from an unusually severe form of migraine, came to Kiholm for treatment. A year or two earlier she had changed over to the Waerland diet and had practically got rid of the migraine and an accompanying dizziness. Before that she had had acute attacks of migraine in the mornings, between four and six o'clock, accompanied by vomiting, unconsciousness, and cramp. During the attacks her face became blue. She had had continual dizziness and severe anemia (45% hem.). Her blood sedimentation rate had been up to 140. When she came to Kiholm her sedimentation rate was still 82 and her blood far from normal.

She was put on a bland diet, raw juices, and cleansing treatment and in a surprisingly short time (because previously she had been for some time on a good diet) the sedimentation rate had gone down to 22 and the hemoglobin had risen to 65%.

Frau Wenger, born in 1891, was one of my patients at Sonnenhof. She had suffered from severe migraine for ten years, hardly a day passing without great pain. Like many people suffering from headaches, she had resorted to narcotics. Her liver was not functioning normally and she had been constipated as long as she could remember.

She was put on a fast and, to her astonishment, the headache was relieved after only three days. It is the usual course for the headache to increase at the beginning of a fast and then, after two or three days, to diminish in intensity or clear up altogether. Excepting high blood pressure and anemia, no symptoms are more rewarding to treat than the various forms of headache.

Frau Wenger continued the cleansing treatment and intermittent fasting for a few weeks and then went home radiantly happy and grateful.

Frau A. Seebach had suffered from migraine for decades. Hers was the typical, one-sided migraine, and the attacks were accompanied by vomiting of bile. In order to carry on her work she took strong caffeine powders, specially made for her. After her gall bladder was removed in 1942, the attacks increased in severity. In November, 1949, she began having feverish attacks, her temperature rising to over 103° and recurring every four weeks with all the usual accompaniments of headache, vomiting, and profuse perspiration. The last few attacks lasted 36 hours. For two years Frau Seebach was unable to work.

In April, 1952, she resumed work but could manage only with the aid of strong injections of morphia. In February, 1953, she changed over to the Waerland diet, which worked wonders for her. In three months the migraine had gone. She began to gain weight and steadily built up her health till she was better than she had ever imagined possible. A typical indication that her body had been cleared of accumulations of waste matter and poisons was that after a time she was able to stand the sun. Most people are unable to expose themselves to strong sunshine, when in a highly toxic condition, without feeling tired and sick or dizzy or having a headache.

For twenty-three years before changing over to the Waerland diet, Frau Seebach had been a vegetarian, i.e., she had lived mostly on cooked vegetables, but in spite of this her condition had only grown steadily worse.

Headaches and smoking

The following two patients were able to overcome the craving for nicotine by means of the Waerland diet.

Herr G. H. had contracted *malaria tropica* during the second world war. His spine had been badly injured and he had had swamp fever. As a consequence of having been buried alive during a bombing attack, he had acute headaches. In order to endure all the physical and mental strain of the war he had become a heavy smoker.

He came as a patient to Elmau and, under protest, was persuaded to fast and to have internal cleansing treatment. After about a week of this the headache began to lessen somewhat in severity. By means of the fast we were able to allay the antibodies against the nicotine, which had accumulated in the body, so that he lost the craving for tobacco.

On returning home after six weeks he felt perfectly well.

Herr F., born in 1917, came to Kiholm in the winter of 1954. He had had a gastric ulcer for many years and two thirds of the stomach had been surgically removed.

His work was very strenuous, and in order to cope with it he had given way to taking phenedrin tablets. This drug acts like a whip on the nervous system, taking away the desire for sleep and disguising fatigue, which is a natural danger signal. Then, one day, the game is up and the whole nervous system collapses, leaving the patient in a state of utter apathy and weakness. If he has also been addicted to nicotine, the collapse is still greater.

Herr F. had been taking as many as thirty tablets a day as well as smoking heavily, and this was the condition in which he arrived at Kiholm. He lay in bed, dead tired but unable to sleep, hungry but unable to assimilate food. His will to live and all pleasure in life were nonexistent and his nervous strength was exhausted.

On account of his ravenous hunger I could not let him fast. He had to eat often, and the meals had to consist of very easily digested alkaline foods which would aid the cleansing process and yet be bland. He was given the appropriate diet for gastric ulcer patients, including decoction plus carrot juice between meals, and we tried to clear out the poisons with enemas and irrigations.

Our task was to get the patient on his legs and out into the fresh air for at least short periods, to increase the circulation of the blood and give it oxygen. Also we had to wean him from the nicotine and other poisonous drugs.

The beginning was difficult and meant repeated persuasion. But as soon as the patient got out of doors and began to move about, the improvement was rapid. It was wonderful to see how the apathy and hopelessness were, within a short time, transformed into cheerfulness and the will to live. Sleep returned and he grew stronger.

Herr F. was, unfortunately, not able to stay with us for more than a few weeks, but when he left he was greatly missed. For he had not only been able to overcome his own physical and mental depression but had progressed so far that he had become a real comfort and source of encouragement to many of the other patients. His joy at having got the better of his craving for tobacco and no longer being dependent upon drugs was touching.

Insomnia

The inability to sleep is one of the commonest results of faulty diet and accumulated waste products. It will almost always disappear when healthful eating and habits of living are introduced. For thirty years I suffered from insomnia and could not sleep for one night without a sleeping pill. But when I changed over to the Waerland diet, I threw away all my medicines and sleep returned in relation to the reduction of toxins in the body. I have since been able to help many victims of insomnia and only remember one case which was not cured.

Sleepless, nervous patients should not fast. Natural sedatives from herbs are often very useful. In Germany we found a homeopathic preparation, *plantival*, excellent for nerve sufferers. In Sweden I replace this by a tea made from equal quantities of salvia, hops, and camomile, taken in bed just before sleep is desired. It is very effective.

The best means of counteracting sleeplessness is a morning walk before breakfast. People who do not sleep well tend to lie abed in the morning, but this is the worst thing possible. The earlier they get up and the longer they are able to extend the walk, the better they will sleep. And when they go to bed at night, they should settle down comfortably and consciously relax, while breathing deeply. The mind should be filled with pleasant memories and scenes, putting aside all restless or gloomy thoughts. They should do the same if they wake up in the night after, perhaps, eating a biscuit or rusk, or some sweet fruit. This draws the blood down from the head to the digestive organs and makes it easier to go to sleep again.

Constipation

It is easy to understand why the Waerland diet, which contains so much cellulose and roughage to encourage peristalsis, is so good for constipation. Fasting and internal cleansing are also most important aids in this as in so many other complaints. Most invalids are constipated. It often takes tremendous patience, energy, and work to get a slack intestine, which has been slowly atrophying for years, to act naturally. One has to resort to colonic irrigation, massage and abdominal exercises, supplemented by herbal teas and decoctions of laxative plants.

Our morning drink, containing linseed and bran (for severe cases also containing figs and prunes soaked overnight), also kruska, all regulate the activity of the bowels. If the constipation is obstinate, psyllium seed or a decoction of frangula bark (buckthorn) may be used. The latter, especially, is excellent, being both mild and effective. It is perfectly harmless and may be continued indefinitely; it is best taken in the morning, but in obstinate cases may also be taken in the evening. To prepare:

Boil the crushed frangula bark (obtainable from a

druggist) for ten minutes in ten times the quantity of water. A little water should be added while boiling to maintain the proportion of one to ten.

I can safely say that thousands of cases of severe constipation have been cured by the Waerland therapy. At the same time it saves people from the unspeakable suffering which follows in the train of constipation.

18 / Anemia, high blood pressure, and disorders of the heart

One of the main reasons why the Waerland diet has such a unique influence on our health is that it raises the hemoglobin content and creates good blood. The blood is the life fluid, nourishing and building up all our organs and cells, and our health depends primarily on its nature and quality.

Millions of people today are living on a diet that not only is deficient in vitamins and minerals but also contains putrefactive elements in large proportions. This diet cannot possibly create good blood. Only fresh, organic foods, containing all the substances needed by the body in building up sound cells, can do this.

Several decades ago the great hospitals in America began to treat acute septic diseases with injections of chlorophyll, which had astonishing results. This treatment has become known all over the world and is often used in treating desperate cases, now that the marvelous blood-forming, regenerative qualities of chlorophyll have been established.

Anemia

Since cholorophyll is admittedly so valuable in nutrition, particularly on account of its influence on the blood formation, why do we so often go the long way round via synthetic preparations, at a time when the resistance of the body is already low, instead of seeing that we get good blood through a natural diet, rich in chlorophyll?

Not even during our cold northern winters do we need to go without chlorophyll. Underneath the snow, even in the most severe cold, kale flourishes, and it replaces all the summer wealth of green stuff. The leaves can be put through a mincer, after removing the coarse parts, and served raw; if desired, the minced kale can be mixed with mashed potato and dressed with sour milk. We may eat the young leaves whole and we may cook the larger leaves until they are tender.

Early in the spring, when there is still a little snow on the ground, the first tender leaves of nettles and dandelions peep out and we can use them. From then on until late autumn there is a wealth of chlorophyll to be found. The tender dandelion leaves can be eaten as salad, and coarser ones can be boiled to make a splendid mineral drink for morning and afternoon. Nettles and dandelions can well be boiled together. The raw juice pressed from dandelion leaves and nettles can be given diluted with juice from root vegetables, or water in which potatoes or other vegetables have been boiled. (These two juices are so concentrated that they should never be taken undiluted.) Tender nettles are delicious, boiled for a few minutes and served with a pat of butter. They can also be chopped raw, mixed with mashed potatoes flavored with herbs or chives, and served with a dressing of sour milk.

Beet juice is excellent for enriching and purifying the

blood. It can be mixed with a half quantity of vegetable water or carrot juice—or with both, one third of each. The beet juice is strongly concentrated and has a rather sharp, acrid taste if grown on artificially fertilized soil.

The wealth of salads and green things the summer offers us is a splendid source of blood-forming elements. But it is not only the green leaf that is so important. Let us, in the spring, when the sap is rising in the tree trunks and the leaves are in bud, bore a hole in the white trunk of the birch tree and gather the purifying elixir of life it offers. Let us drink a glass of the excellent birch sap each day for a couple of weeks. And let us, besides, if the heart permits, go on a fast in the springtime, when all the life forces are rising. The phenomenal health of the people of the Hunza is, to a large extent, due to the long, enforced fast they undergo every spring. It is the best time for fasting.

The air we breathe is of the greatest importance in the formation of blood, and we should see to it that our air is fully charged with oxygen by keeping the windows open night and day and living out of doors as much as possible. Close, used-up air, laden with tobacco smoke and other injurious gases, hinders the functioning of our bodies just as badly as the wrong kind of food.

Exercise in the fresh air is absolutely essential to health, in order to stimulate the circulation and the combustion of waste matter. If we make full use of all these health factors and the rich store of life-giving elements in the plant world, our blood will be regenerated and become the inexhaustible well of life from which our cells and organs can draw their sustenance and their strength.

When we realize this, it is little wonder that so many people living on commercialized, devitalized foods no longer have sound blood. It is just as understandable that the Waerland therapies and the Waerland diet, rich in chlorophyll, restore the blood to normal. Again and again I have observed a surprisingly quick regeneration of the blood, even in severe cases of leukemia.

In cases of serious blood diseases it is an excellent thing if the patient can stay for a time in high mountain air, where the red corpuscles increase more rapidly. In certain severe cases I have given the patients a supplementary course of Vitamin B_{12}. When the disease has reached a certain stage, all the natural means of stimulating the formation of blood must be resorted to.

High blood pressure

This is, perhaps, modern disorder number one and is, unfortunately, very widely regarded as incurable. Nevertheless it is being reduced more easily and completely than any other trouble, by means of a natural, fully adequate diet.

The very large number of cases we have treated go to prove that this disorder, like so many others, is actually brought on by an unnatural way of living and a diet which causes, or encourages, toxicity in the body.

If we live on a biologically wrong diet, the blood stream

becomes flooded with the waste products of metabolism, which impede its passage through the blood vessels and eventually cause cramp in the capillaries. In order to press the blood forward through the partially blocked vessels, the heart increases its pressure. When, however, the body is relieved of all unnecessary accumulations of waste products, the blood pressure is automatically reduced.

The cleansing of the organism is achieved in the usual way, either by fasting or on a limited, alkaline diet. At the same time the work of the excretory organs must be supported in every way possible by drinking plenty of fluid and by means of enemas.

Younger patients with good heart action can begin at once with a fast on raw alkaline juices (see p. 200).

After the fast has been broken, when the blood pressure in most cases has become normal, the patient should continue for a time on the limited diet (see p. 201).

All patients with high blood pressure who are unable to fast, owing to heart weakness, should begin the cure on the limited diet.

Cases of excessive weight also respond very well to this limited diet, losing up to twelve or fourteen pounds in two weeks.

The limited diet may be continued for a month or two. Here, as in all other cases, the treatment must be individual for each patient. If a sensation of weakness should be felt, this will be due to excessive alkalinity of the blood. This is harmless and passes quickly. An addition of one or two slices of bread to the daily dietary at once restores the natural balance between acids and alkalies in the blood. Patients can arrange periodic semi-fasts on the limited diet, alternating with periods on the ordinary Waerland diet.

Disorders of the heart

Excellent results have also been achieved in the treatment of heart troubles, even in long-standing cases of great severity where strong drugs have been used previously. After a little time we have always been able to discard the strong drugs and use instead a more gentle, homeopathic strengthening remedy for the heart, which will build up the weakened muscle. Tincture of crataegus is the remedy I have found most efficacious, given in a dosage of five drops morning and evening or, in slighter cases, only in the morning. This remedy can never do harm and does not lose its effect even over long periods.

Heart patients cannot as a rule stand the effort of fasting. In such cases we recommend a semi-fast, or the limited diet already described. The usual cleansing treatment must of course be given. When the body is freed from waste matter and toxins, the heart is relieved and has a chance to rest and be regenerated.

It is a joy to see how the patients liven up as the cleansing of the body proceeds. They begin to move in quite a different way, going up and down stairs and out for walks. The heart attacks, breathlessness, and pains disappear very rapidly in most cases.

An overstrained or diseased heart is not able to stand the drinking of large quantities of fluid at a time. Great care must therefore be taken at first and the fluid intake reduced to a little more than half the usual quantity, i.e., to about one quart daily, divided into three separate drinks. The patient must drink very slowly, in sips, and never take cold drinks i.e., under body temperature. He should try by degrees to drink more, as it is of paramount importance that the excretory organs should function properly. The success of the cleansing processes depends on this.

A heart patient should never overexert himself. Nevertheless, he should slowly train himself to take walks and carefully exercise his muscles. The circulation of the blood must be stimulated in every way, e.g., by dry brushing of the skin, massage, and cold sponging. Each limb in turn should be sponged over with water as cold as possible and immediately dried with a rough towel. The dry brushing then follows, with great vigor, until the skin is warm and glowing.

Carbonic-acid baths are very beneficial, and after improvement has begun, alternating hot-and-cold baths for the feet and arms will help.

Resting by an open window and in a reclining chair out of doors are also part of the cure. Heart patients need fresh air day and night. Plenty of oxygen is at least as important as a healthy diet.

The diet should contain all essential elements of proper nutrition and yet be light: no large portions of kruska, no cheese except cottage, or goat's-milk (whey) cheese, and not much butter. Rawkost; fruit and sour milk; potatoes and molino; potato porridge (a little sweet milk and slightly sweetened stewed fruit with the porridge); crisp bread and an occasional slice of wholemeal bread—all these are suitable. If the patient's digestion can tolerate onions and garlic, these are extremely valuable in heart cases. The chief thing to remember is that every meal should be moderate, with no very large portions of any food. Heart sufferers should be slim and light in weight, each superfluous pound being a further burden on the heart. Vitamins B and E are important aids and should be taken for some time, in the form of yeast and wheat-germ oil. Heart patients should also take a little honey every day.

The following cases are encouraging:

Herr K. was a patient of mine at Bad Soden in the autumn of 1953. For seven years he had had valvular trouble, following pneumonia, and had been having daily injections of strophanthus. He had edema badly and felt extremely weak and ill, constantly troubled by severe heart attacks, having to stay in bed most of the time.

In the month during which he underwent treatment at Haus Alice, he made great progress. The attacks became less severe and the intervals between them longer. He was soon able to get up and take short walks, gradually increasing the distance. His general condition showed a marked improvement and the paralyzing hopelessness was gone.

Frau B. came as a patient to Elmau, having three years previously damaged her heart muscle. The muscle was still very weak and she had been in bed for six weeks before coming to Elmau. She, also, had treatment for one month, during which the heart muscle recovered very quickly. The patient left us radiantly grateful, and when I saw her again, about a year later, I hardly knew her. She was then the picture of health.

Frau G. was another patient at Elmau. She was suffering from cramp in the coronary arteries, circulatory disturbances, and inflammation of the lymph glands. She had chronic constipation, varicose veins, and certain troubles connected with the menopause. Her general condition was poor and she had fits of acute depression as a result of the constipation.

The varicose veins were successfully treated with cabbage compresses; the limited diet, internal cleansing and tincture of crataegus worked wonders. After a month, a happy, radiant patient went home with newly won health.

Herr F. was treated at Elmau for angina pectoris, which had started twenty-four years earlier. Four years after the onset of this illness he suffered a complete breakdown. A series of cures and periods of treatment at sanatoria had given temporary relief, but in 1949 his condition had seriously worsened. One month's treatment at Elmau made a new man of him.

Frau McNeil came to Elmau from Hildesheim to thank me for the wonderful health she had gained through the Waerland diet. She was twenty-nine years old and had been saved by the change of diet from long-standing hopeless suffering. At the early age of twelve her thyroid gland had begun to swell. At eighteen she had an enlarged heart, and severe, painful attacks. She had never felt well.

Then she married. When she was pregnant a large

blood tumor formed in the uterine passage and had to be surgically removed. Her life was miserable. She was so weak that she could not go upstairs or do any work and she never went out. Her heart was always inadequate.

After the change of diet her whole life had changed. She felt newborn and her strength and spirits rose day by day. She began to go in for outdoor pursuits and finally she, who had not had strength even to go upstairs, won first prize in a swimming competition and another prize for a type of skiing known as *slalom.** No one could have imagined that so much suffering lay behind her as she sat opposite me, full of health and vitality.

Frau B., until a few years before I met her, was bedridden with very high blood pressure. Her condition was regarded as incurable and very grave. She was taken to a hospital, where she asked if there was no special diet she might try for her complaint. The reply was that diet had not the slightest effect on her condition.

Having in vain tried all that this great modern hospital had to offer, she had herself discharged and, at home, changed over to the Waerland diet. Her condition improved rapidly and she was soon able to get up. It was not long before she was able to do her own housework.

After a time, she rang up the hospital and asked if she might come to have her blood pressure checked. The head doctor was surprised that she was able to go to him. He was still more surprised when he examined her and found that her blood pressure was normal. When she told him about her change of diet, he said with some embarrass-

* See Glossary.

ment: "Well, if only I had known that you were able to take *rawkost* . . ." When Frau B. asked him to explain his former opinion the doctor was silent.

Frau D. E., of St. Gallen, writes: "I, too, have experienced the miracle that can be wrought by a change of diet and living. And it is only a year since I made the change. I wish I had known at least ten years sooner about your diet and way of living; I should then have been spared much suffering. We cannot alter the past, of course, and I am grateful that through making the change I saved myself from a premature death. That was the threat overhanging my children and me.

"Ever since I was eighteen I had suffered from valvular heart trouble. Later, heart neurosis and muscular changes were added. I often had severe heart attacks, particularly when a certain wind was blowing (this wind, a southerly gale coming from Africa, is called sirocco, or föhn, in the countries of Southern Europe and has a very unpleasant effect on sensitive people). I also had severe migraine at these times, with unbearable pain.

"The headaches disappeared soon after the change of diet, and the heart attacks were less severe and not so frequent. I no longer feel the effect of the föhn, which had upset me for thirty years. The druggists have lost a good customer in me as I used to live on pills and powders to steady my heart and numb the pain. That time is now past. I cannot understand that such a change could take place in such a short time—I could never have dreamt it was possible. Another thing is that the recurrent nettle-rash which I have had since I was twenty, has gone. It was my fine complexion that first gave my people something to think about.

"My initiative has also come back. For many years I was unable to go out in the evenings owing to my weak heart, but now for the last year I have been going to the theater quite often, also to lectures and the cinema. It is such a joy to be no longer afraid of attacks and breakdowns. For many years I was unable to travel at all, but now I can go wherever I like once more.

"Life has opened up again for me and I am infinitely happy and grateful for the inestimable gift of health."

19 / Goitre

Simple goitre is most prevalent in districts where the soil is deficient in iodine. It is, therefore, primarily a deficiency disease. Whenever a vital element is lacking in the organism, the inward equilibrium, so finely balanced by nature, is disturbed, and adverse changes take place. In the case of goitre it is the activity of the glands which has been upset. The thyroid gland, which is vitally important for all the functions of the body, since it is one of the regulators of metabolism, becomes swollen through strain and is no longer able to fulfil its purpose.

There are two types of goitre, one ("simple goitre") where the swelling is outward and the other, more dangerous, which swells inwardly. The latter type is known as exophthalmic goitre, or Graves' or Basedow's disease, and often causes choking symptoms.

The lack of iodine is not the only cause of goitre. It is often the end result of a slowly accumulating toxicity in the organism, which has gradually disorganized the activity of the thyroid gland. Iodine deficiency is, however, one of the main causes, and that is why goitre usually occurs in particular districts and is more prevalent in Switzerland and the mountains of Southern Germany, where the soil is lacking in this vital element, than in the Scandinavian countries.

Goitre is a protracted and very obstinate disease, but the fact that severe and even "hopeless" cases can be cured will be seen from the instances described in this chapter. The road to health goes, as in other diseases, by way of a cleansing, alkaline diet. Unfortunately, many goitre patients cannot stand a fast and, this short cut being blocked, it takes longer to detoxicate the body. A fast can produce a very adverse reaction in a goitre patient, but here, as in all things, the exception proves the rule.

Goitre patients with *overactive* thyroid gland (exophthalmic type) are generally very thin. The metabolism proceeds too quickly and they suffer from continuous hunger which cannot be satisfied, however much they eat. It is almost impossible for them to increase in weight.

Entirely different symptoms indicate the *insufficient activity* of the thyroid gland. A fast can be carried out and there are no unnatural sensations of hunger nor the extreme thinness. Most goitre patients suffer from insomnia, nervousness, and depression. Usually there has been longstanding constipation with accompanying chronic poisoning of the organism, which has been the starting point of the trouble.

Goitre patients should live on the ordinary Waerland diet. If they come from a district where there is iodine deficiency, they should have a daily supplementary dose of it by taking the Japanese seaweed, so rich in iodine, known as agar-agar. One or two tablespoons of finely cut agar-agar in the morning drink or chewed, dry, before meals, will be sufficient. There are other iodine preparations obtainable at drugstores or health-food stores, in most countries, varying with available supplies; but they should always be in *natural form,* i.e., not in the form of extracts or mixed with chemicals. To relieve nervousness, sedative teas can be given, such as valerian tea. Relaxation exercises and deep breathing morning and evening, and at midday, are very important.

I hope that sufferers from goitre will gain fresh courage from the following descriptions of the battle of two Swedish athletes against this dread disease, and their success.

Karl Widmark, a barber and hairdresser by profession, was a keen athlete, living in the town of Västeras. He had been delicate from childhood but through his energy and keenness succeeded in becoming a top-rank sportsman. He went in for skiing and canoeing and eventually became a member of the Aros Troupe, one of Sweden's most famous gymnastic and athletic teams. In 1924 he had won the district championship in paddling and continued to improve until, in 1935, he was regarded as a certainty for the Olympic Games in Berlin the following year. But his health failed him during the training period and he was overcome by great weakness, sleeplessness, and loss of appetite. In spite of persistent effort he broke down, the doctor diagnosing complete breakdown of the nervous system, incurable heart disease, and exophthalmic goitre.

After a year of all kinds of treatments, including X-ray,

drugs, and injections, at his local hospital, he was no better and was so depressed by the tragedy of his broken career that he was contemplating suicide when, in the summer of 1936, Are Waerland returned to Sweden. The story of how Waerland had transformed himself from a human wreck into a strong man gave Widmark fresh hope. Just at that time the *Frisksport Magazine* published an invitation to join in a nutrition experiment which was to last for three years, the results to be recorded and to be a test of the validity of the Waerland ideas on health and diet.*

To Karl Widmark, the idea that his own troubles might have been caused by mistakes in living and a diet which had gradually broken down his health was completely new. He read the invitation and, having nothing to lose, said he might try. He enrolled for the experiment and very soon had the surprise of his life. In three months he was able to resume his training and, during the next winter and spring, took part in skiing and track competitions, improving in health all the time. He had to go carefully at first, but steadily found he could do more and more. At the end of a year he was in better health than ever.

These excellent results were due to his indomitable energy and the consistency and endurance with which he carried out the new system of diet and daily living. He

* About 1,300 people of all classes and occupations faithfully carried out this experiment and were known as "The Sun Vikings." All of them attained better health than they had ever known was possible. Their diet is described in Chap. 3.

adopted the Waerland diet in its strictest and simplest form, drinking plenty of fluids to ensure that the bowels did their part in the fundamental cleansing process and rid the body of all toxins and accumulated waste matter. Every morning he rose early enough to take a cold bath (in winter he rolled in the snow), then gave his skin a good dry brushing and went out for an hour's vigorous exercise in the fresh air before breakfast.

By the summer of 1938 he was in top form and entered the international canoe races at Vaxholm, Sweden. The foreign entrants were numerous. The Austrian Olympic winner, Hradetzki, was regarded generally as certain to be champion. Karl Widmark, the hairdresser who had newly recovered from a severe illness, was Sweden's best man, being now a well-trained, sun-tanned sportsman.

And Karl Widmark was the great sensation of the competition. He won the two most important canoe races, the one-kilometer and the ten-kilometer, in each case reaching the goal far ahead of all the others. This made him world champion.

Lester Larson was another young Swedish sportsman who made a wonderful recovery from the same disease. At the age of twenty he developed exophthalmic goitre. In the autumn of 1943, after three months' treatment in a hospital, his case was regarded as hopeless. He was unable to stand, his heart was weak and irregular, his eyes protruded, and his hands trembled so much that he could not eat without help.

As a last attempt to save his life, an operation was decided on. All preparations were made and Larson lay on the operating table; but when injected with a sedative prior to the general anesthetic, alarming symptoms of paralysis arose. The operation had to be abandoned and he was taken into a small private room reserved for hopeless cases. The doctors had given up hope.

But when the need is greatest, help is at hand. In this desperate condition Larson was visited by a friend who was a Waerlandist. He had cured himself of a serious illness and afterward helped many others back to health. He now succeeded in arousing a spark of interest in the almost dying Larson. Perhaps, he thought, even for him there might be hope. It would be worth trying to follow his friend's advice. In spite of the protests of his family and the doctors, Lester Larson made a momentous decision; he left the hospital and went to stay with his friend. This caused a tremendous commotion and everybody expected him to die. Everybody, that is, except the friend who had decided to try to save his life.

There now followed a thorough internal cleansing. Larson had been a keen football player, playing in important matches and apparently leading a healthy life, but he had suffered from constipation for many years and had lived on a diet which offered no help in this respect, while it undoubtedly contributed to the accumulation of waste matter in the tissues.

The alkaline *rawkost*, raw juices, herb teas, and enemas set all the natural processes of elimination to work and an amazing quantity of impurities was cleaned out. Even the mucous membrane of the nose and throat helped the good work along by excretions of phlegm and mucus.

The patient had always had a bad complexion, with spots and eczema, but these gradually disappeared. He had also had a polyp in the nose and had breathed through his mouth as long as he could remember. His friend bought sticking plaster and sealed his mouth at night so that he was obliged to breathe through his nose. The consequence was that it became easier and easier until the nostrils were clear and breathing through the nose became spontaneous.

The swelling in the thyroid gland went down and the bowels functioned better. When the stools had become odorless and of the right consistency, the enemas were discontinued. The patient gradually grew stronger and his eyes went back into their sockets. Finally the day came when the thyroid gland had resumed its natural size and normal function.

In the middle of January, 1944, Lester Larson went back to his work and, two weeks later, he played in a football match. It had taken only a little over three months to rebuild his health. The new diet and daily living had, in this short time, been the means of overcoming a disease which had brought him to the brink of the grave.

Both Lester Larson and Karl Widmark told their stories of recovery in small pamphlets at the time, which has enabled me to describe these cases in detail. Other cases of goitre have passed through my care, many of them reaching full health, although none has been so dramatic as those of the two young athletes.

Mrs. Martha W. had had four miscarriages and undergone a major internal operation, after which she developed exophthalmic goitre. Through a change to the Waerland diet she became perfectly well.

Mrs. B.O. had been operated on for goitre in 1941. She was still suffering from attacks of suffocating breathlessness when she was admitted to our sanatorium, and had had heart trouble for six years. She also suffered from vertigo. Her blood pressure was very low and she was weak and unable to sleep.

Owing to the state of her heart she was unable to fast but was put on the *limited diet.* Tincture of crataegus was given to strengthen the heart, and also plantival, a homeopathic herbal preparation to help her sleep. She also had tea made from mistletoe.

The result of our treatment and change of diet, combined with cleansing by enemas, was that a marked improvement was established in two weeks.

20 / *Varicose veins, leg ulcers, abscesses, sinusitis*

Varicose veins

In most cases it has been found that a change of diet is sufficient to reduce inflammation of the veins without any other particular treatment. We often hear of cases where the clearing up of the veins has been incidental to a change-over for some other reason. In certain long-standing, severe cases the distention of the veins does not disappear, but all pain and discomfort is eliminated and the diseased condition arrested.

Swelling of the legs is a common symptom where there are varicose veins, because of the sluggish circulation. The passage through the inflamed veins is partially, sometimes completely, blocked so that the blood stream has to find a way through the smaller veins. To counteract this, it is a good thing to raise the foot of the bed at night by placing a pillow under the mattress, or blocks of wood under the legs of the bed, so that the veins more easily empty themselves. If the legs are badly swollen it is necessary to wear an elastic stocking, or bandage. Homeopathic hamamelis (witch hazel) preparations are useful in such cases.

The best remedy for varicose veins we have found is

the cabbage compress (see p. 196). These compresses are most efficacious in all kinds of inflammation. The savoy cabbage is the best, but white cabbage is a good substitute. The cabbage leaves have the capacity of drawing out unhealthy fluids and so arrest the inflammation. The leaves remain effective as long as they are green and fresh, but they must be changed as soon as they wilt and lose color.

Ulceration of the legs

Even very old ulcers, constantly recurring and apparently unhealable, have been healed at our sanatoria through fasting and cleansing treatment—even when the surrounding tissues seemed atrophied and dead. The following case is typical:

Mrs. R., an old countrywoman from Lötschental, came to us at Sonnenhof, our sanatorium on Lake Thun. Her varicose veins had begun decades before and gradually worsened until her legs were ulcerated. In spite of hospital treatment her condition deteriorated until one leg was discolored, bluish-black, and covered with mattery ulcers. The doctors thought amputation would be inevitable.

Mrs. R. lived in a remote village in the mountains. The local priest had heard of our system and what it was doing for all kinds of diseases, and he suggested that she should see what it might do for her. After some hesitation she consented and he brought her to Sonnenhof in his car.

From an orthodox medical point of view her case was hopeless. She had been bedridden for some time, her heart was strained and weak. She had vertigo and a great deal of pain. She had been constipated for many years and was very stout, with watery tissues. Her condition was so serious, and the prospect of improvement so small, that I decided to nurse her myself.

This old peasant woman had never heard of an enema. She did not understand the importance of fasting. It cost her many bitter tears to surrender to all the strange new things that were demanded of her.

First of all she was given a camomile bath (see p. 197) to disinfect the ulcers on her legs. Then we began at once with fasting and cleansing. For her heart she had tincture of crataegus and hamamelis for her veins. As a sedative we gave her plantival and, at night, our sleeping tea of hops, salvia and camomile. She was able to fast in the usual way on raw alkaline juices. Her hard, shapeless legs were raised on a pillow and shielded by a wire cradle to take the weight of the bedclothes.

From the beginning her legs were dressed with cabbage compresses and, as the bad leg was cold and numb, I had to pack it warmly with hot-water bottles. The cabbage leaves drew out much of the unhealthy fluids and withered up in an hour or two. For the first few days they had to be changed every few hours; after a week they lasted longer and a few days later were still fresh after twelve hours.

I now realized that the cabbage leaves had done their part and we must change to another type of compress—

raw onion—to disinfect the ulcers. The patient, whose weak heart made fasting difficult, was now put on the *limited diet.* That meant that she had only *rawkost* and raw juices, supplemented with a little sour milk, a little potato, cottage cheese, and rheumatic bread, which is baked of raw vegetables and potatoes. We continued with the enemas, which were assisted by a mild herbal laxative. Twice a week the patient had a camomile bath.

There is no remedy more antiseptic and healing than the onion. During the first world war the doctors in Russia used this simple remedy for gangrene and suppurating sores with results unequaled up to that time. After only a couple of days, mortifying, putrid sores were quickly healed. In cases where amputation had seemed inevitable, it became unnecessary.

I have had the same experience during my years of practice. It is not even necessary to place the onion directly upon the sore if it is likely to irritate it. The healing, antiseptic radiations from the onion will still be effective if the dressing is laid close to the ulcer, providing the adjacent tissues are still relatively sound.

Mrs. R. had no areas of healthy tissue left on her leg where the onion poultice could be placed, the whole leg being covered with ulcers. The gauze would have stuck and prevented healing. The problem was how to get the onion poultice on to her leg. Finally I placed a long, hard pillow beside the leg, *raised a little above it,* then, from surgical gauze, I made a long, narrow bag and filled it with chopped onion. This was attached to the upper edge of the pillow with large tacking stitches so that it hung just over the leg without touching it. In this way all the ulcers received the radiation from the onions.

Gauze must always be used for onion compresses, and they should be changed every four hours during the daytime. At night the dressings are not renewed unless the patient happens to wake up. Sleep is the best of healers, so one never wakes a patient if it can be avoided.

When we stopped the comforting cabbage compresses and the patient's legs lay uncovered under the protecting cradle, the pains became unbearable. Mrs. R. had always tried to relieve them with damp heat and she was terribly upset by the new method of treatment. It was, however, essential to start the process of healing and the forming of scabs, so the leg had to lie uncovered and dry under the antiseptic rays of the raw onions. We had to struggle through two difficult days until the worst of the pain subsided and the sores began to dry up and heal.

Mrs. R. was soon able to spend several hours each day on the terrace in a reclining chair. The healing went on more quickly. In four weeks the scabs loosened and, where the ulcers had been, all one could see were cleanly healed depressions in the skin. No longer black and blue, the leg was almost natural in color and the patient was able to stand and even walk about a little. Happy and grateful, the old woman returned to her home.

Dr. W., a schoolmaster aged forty-eight, had spent many years in the hospital following a war wound in his thigh. He had undergone many operations for abscesses on the bone and in the muscle tissue. After the last operation at the University Clinic in H., the surgeon had told him that he would be obliged to give up his profession as a teacher and the best thing he could do was to get a wheel chair and find some other means of passing the time. He would, in any case, be obliged to have two further operations every year. This had been the case for several years and nothing different was to be expected.

This verdict made the invalid and his wife think. They decided to try new methods and, above all, to make a change in his diet and manner of living. Sooner than they could have imagined, there was a turn for the better.

Only the old leg ulcers would not heal until cabbage compresses were tried. These brought out copious suppuration at first, but after several weeks the sores healed.

Dr. W.'s vitality and capacity to work increased so much that after a time he no longer thought about taking care of his leg. He worked in his garden and built an addition to his house. For several years his former misery was forgotten.

In the summer of 1953 Dr. W. and his family visited relatives in Lüneburger Heide. Believing that he was now in full health, he thought it no longer necessary to be so careful with his diet, and for six weeks he lived on the same food as his relations, who had rich country meals. A couple of weeks later, after all those years, the leg ulcers broke out again and soon he had inflammation in a vein in his eye, which might have cost him his sight. He returned to the Waerland methods and began a fast on raw juices. In this way he soon arrested the inflammation of the eye and restored his sight. His general condition also improved.

Nevertheless, he had a deep-seated abscess which had to be operated on. It was a bad infection and the surgeon feared it might mean amputation. Happily, his fears were not justified, as the body had thrown out its unwholesome fluids via the abscess and the fast and the cleansing treatment had done their part; suddenly, the sores began to heal.

The surgeon, who had already seen similar unusual healing capacity in other Waerlandists, had to admit: "These people do heal up wonderfully. I have never seen anything like it. It must be their diet."

Sinusitis

External suppurations are much more easily healed than septic conditions which have no outlet, such as certain forms of sinusitis. And yet we have found our treatment effective in most cases of suppuration in the nasal cavities. Only in cases where the pus was entirely enclosed in a bony cavity has an operation been necessary. When the local condition has once cleared up, there is no need to fear the relapses which are so common in these complaints as long as the diet is consistently adhered to. Unsuitable food, with the inevitable accompanying surplus of waste matter in the organism, encourages continual recurrence of the suppurative processes.

The only way to a permanent cure is a change-over to natural foods and, of course, as an initial step, a fasting and cleansing cure. In this way the body will be rid of all waste products, which will be carried off by the organs of elimination in the normal way, and the source of the suppurations will dry up.

The following is an example of a severe case of sinusitis. *Helene H.*, a young girl, developed a purulent infection in all the sinuses, following scarlet fever, and underwent repeated operations. In addition, she had meningitis, septicemia, and double pleurisy. For three months she hovered between life and death. When at last she was out of danger, her heart was seriously impaired and she had to lie in bed for several months.

For several years afterwards she had frequent recurrences of the sinus infections, which involved painful treatments. Then, for a whole year, a suppurating boil at the root of the nose reduced her to a state of extreme debility.

When she was nineteen, she thought she would like to try natural healing but leaned toward a system less radical than the Waerland method. So we took her to Switzerland, to a sanatorium where the food was a compromise between the ordinary, civilized diet and our stricter, mainly raw, lacto-vegetarian diet, fortunately becoming more widely used among food reformers. She carried out the instructions conscientiously for several weeks but, in spite of this, her condition became worse and we had to consult a specialist in Zürich. His verdict was alarming. He had found that the dividing wall between the frontal sinuses was already worn through, so that there was danger that the pus would spread to the brain. He considered that four big operations would be necessary, entailing at least six months in the hospital.

When we left the consulting room I begged Helene to give our diet a trial for four weeks under my direction. If in this time no improvement was evident, she would have to undergo the operations. She agreed and we left Zürich together and went to Ascona, in the province of Tessin. There, in the beautiful Monte Verita hotel, she was able to obtain an excellent Waerland diet.

On arrival at Ascona she was pale, listless, and weak, with no apparent interest in life. At first she had no appetite, but soon the new diet began to taste better and it was not long before she was actually enjoying her food. The color came back to her cheeks and her eyes grew clearer. She awoke as if from a nightmare, and as her vitality increased she grew livelier every day. The suppuration from the boil at the root of her nose dwindled and finally ceased, and the opening healed up.

Helene was quite transformed and joined in walks and excursions with wholehearted enjoyment.

After four weeks she was examined by a specialist and her sinuses X-rayed. The doctor said: "There must be some mistake. Severe sinusitis like that could not possibly heal in such a short time. Certainly it is perfectly obvious that there has been an acute condition with copious suppuration, but the scars indicate that it must have cleared up quite a long time ago."

Such an experience is vouchsafed only to the new art of healing in closest harmony with the eternal laws of nature, and in co-operation with the healing forces inherent in the body itself.

21 / *The value of correct breathing*

All life is inexorably dependent upon breathing. To breathe is to live: without breathing there is no life. From the first breath of the newborn babe to the last sigh of the dying man, the flame of life is kept burning by the unbroken rhythm of the breath. Breathing is, thus, just about the most important of all the functions of the body, upon which all its other physical manifestations are dependent. A man can live a long time without eating, a shorter time without drinking, but only a few minutes without breathing.

In order to live a healthy life, free from disease and with undiminished vitality, it is necessary not only to breathe but to breathe in the right way. Conscious control of our breathing prolongs our life and increases our vitality, while careless, neglected breathing shortens life, lowers the vitality, and prepares the ground for infections.

This is one of the ways in which modern life has led us into unnatural, injurious habits. We have paid a high price for civilization. Primitive races, not yet affected by our unnatural ways of living, still breathe in a natural manner. Only a small percentage of all civilized peoples breathe correctly. The results are evident in rounded shoulders, sunken chests, the increasing incidence of diseases of the respiratory organs, and the advance of tuberculosis.* Some well-known authorities have pointed out that a single generation of people who breathed correctly could regenerate the whole of our race. Many scientists of East and West recognize that correct breathing and health are inseparable.

The greatest fault in the breathing of most people these days is that the lungs are only partially filled. Their breathing is shallow, filling only the top part of the lungs, leaving stale air in the lower part. The expression "take a deep breath" is often used humorously, referring to the need for some special effort, mental or physical, in facing up to an unusual situation, but it is scientifically correct. Deep breathing supplies the blood with the greatest possible amount of oxygen. A sensation of warmth, vitality, and ease fills the whole of our being when the lungs work in a natural, effective manner. In correct breathing the movements of the diaphragm also act as a gentle massage of the abdominal organs and stimulate their functions.

The importance of breathing is being more widely recognized, and there are many good systems of training for those who need to relearn this natural function. It is wise to study a simple book on breathing† or to take some lessons from an expert rather than merely to begin taking "deep breaths." It is a science which requires a knowledge of the structure of the organs involved; unwise, over-

* Mrs. Waerland believes that tuberculosis is increasing, although mortality from it is decreasing.

† Recommended: *The Science of Breath* by Yogi Ramacharaka.

energetic breathing, especially at first, may do more harm than good. One "safe" exercise is to expel, gently and without strain, all the air in the lungs as far as possible. The natural intake will follow without effort, filling the lungs with fresh air.

Singing is another way of cultivating good breathing. It is not necessary to have a wonderful voice. Try to sing a long note, then a series of notes, then a tune—you will be surprised how fascinating it is and how invigorating.

How often the stone which is rejected is, in reality, the cornerstone of the temple of health. We try to maintain our health by complicated cures and treatments instead of taking the straight, simple way of nature. If only we followed the natural laws of our body, letting each organ function in the right way, making use of all the wonderful possibilities of development and regeneration, the human race could look forward into a healthier, happier future.

22 / *Conclusion: The mental and spiritual*

And so . . . I see them as they pass before my mind's eye, a long line of suffering humanity. Weary and downcast they came. With renewed hope and returning health, often completely cured, they went back to their homes.

What happiness it is to work in harmony with the healing forces of nature, to see one disease after another being overcome by natural food and natural methods of treatment, to see the brightness return to sad eyes and deep depression give way to a new *joie de vivre.*

Life is great and glorious, full of wonders and surprises. We must never give up, believing that for us there is no longer any help. As long as there is a spark of the sacred flame of life still left in a tortured human shell, we must not lose hope. *For where there is life there is hope.*

This book describes natural, health-building methods of treatment: fasting, internal cleansing, diet, fresh air, massage, and baths—all of which are important for the restoration of health to our bodies—but health is not created by physical means alone. The most important thing of all is our inward attitude toward everything we encounter in life, not least our difficulties and our bodily ills. A positive outlook is the main factor in mental and physical health.

If we use the creative forces within us to transform the negative things that confront us into positive values, we cannot fail to be strengthened and deepened. One who has passed through the fire of acute mental or physical pain and emerged triumphant is able to draw strength and richness from the well of suffering. He will also be able to imbue others with the hope and light kindled in his own soul. It is the greatest of a physician's tasks to arouse in his patient fresh courage and confidence, new energy and the will to live. If he succeeds in this, miracles will happen. The healer is privileged to be an instrument of the divine creative forces all around us and in nature. He should be able to radiate his own positive outlook, acting as a channel for the Life Force to the one in whom it is burning low.

The love of life is a tremendous power in overcoming disease. If we are animated by a strong life urge, we shall be armed and able to conquer all negative, disease-producing influences. We, ourselves, can awaken and foster positive thoughts in our minds. We can create and control our own moods. As the years pass, we can develop our inward powers and our self-control. We were not born to be the slaves of a capricious fate but to become purposeful, free, and harmonious personalities.

We are collaborators in an unending act of creation. We have been given the stuff from which to shape our lives, but the most valuable material is often the most difficult to handle.

All this would be an impossible task for us if we had to carry it out alone and on our own strength. We could achieve nothing without a contact with the Divine Source of power. Unless we open our hearts and minds to the Universal Father and receive the blessing of God on all our strivings and longings, they will be barren and futile. This inward preparedness is something in which we can train ourselves. The cultivation of a quiet mind, an inward stillness, opens the way for us to contact the divine creative and healing forces; and if we dedicate the whole of our will, our desires, and our longing to this end, we can develop our gifts and set our lives in a right direction.

However helpless and weak we feel, we must not despair. We must not grow weary of living in a state of inward preparedness, of being ready to open ourselves to all the vitalizing streams of power. Every seeking soul has access to them, and it depends upon ourselves whether we are able to receive them.

A positive acceptance of our life material, confidence and faith in a divine purpose, a thankful heart and the love of life are the true foundations for a sound mind in a sound body.

23 / *Recipes and instructions*

Beanskin tea

Allow 1 heaping tablespoonful of bean pods to 2 cups of water (4 deciliters). Put the bean pods in hot water to soak overnight and boil next morning for 10 minutes. Diabetic patients usually have bean-pod tea four times a day. The quantity required for the day should be made in the morning.

Bread for rheumatism

(To be given to rheumatic patients, patients with eczema, diabetics, and all who are excessively acid and unable, therefore, to tolerate wholemeal bread.)

Take equal parts of *raw vegetables* (carrots, beets, celeriac, fennel, cabbage, parsley, dandelion leaves, nettles, etc.) and cold *boiled potatoes;* add *wholemeal* (preferably home ground) and *bran.* The vegetables can be varied and mixed according to taste and availability.

Put the vegetables through a grinder with the unpeeled boiled potatoes. Finely chopped flavoring herbs may be added. Work in the flour until the right consistency is obtained—a soft dough—and then roll out as thin as possible on a board strewn with bran. Cut into rounds with a pastry cutter, or a cup, and dry the rounds on an electric hot plate or a baking tin on top of the stove. They must not be dried too slowly or with too-great heat or they will be tough. Turn during the drying process.

Rheumatic bread does not keep and must, therefore, be used on the day it is baked. Potatoes boiled the same day should be used and the vegetables be fresh and juicy.

Cabbage compresses

The best kind of cabbage to use is the Savoy, but if this is not available, ordinary cabbage can be used.

Choose the greenest, juiciest leaves and, after cutting away the thick, coarse veins, wash the leaves in *warm* water and dry with a towel. (The compress must not be applied cold or wet.) Then roll the leaves out flat with a rolling pin or a large bottle, until they are soft and pliable and as smooth as possible.

Arrange the leaves smoothly, overlapping each other like tiles on a roof, over the affected part. Lumps and creases may cause pain. For small areas, the leaves can be cut in thin strips. Lay a handkerchief, towel, or linen cloth next the cabbage and over that a pad of wadding or soft woolen cloth, finally securing the whole with an elastic bandage. The compress may well be kept on all day or all night without being changed. For patients in bed, the compress should be changed morning and evening and, once a day, the affected part should be washed with a decoction of camomile. If, however, the leaves wither or change color, they must be replaced by fresh ones more frequently.

Calcium treatment for tuberculosis

Place 2 eggs in a china bowl with the juice of four lemons. Then put the bowl in a cool place and cover with a plate. Turn the eggs every other day. After six days the lemon juice will have drawn the calcium out of the eggs and they can be thrown away. The patient takes 2 tablespoonfuls of the juice every day. Every third day two more eggs are laid in lemon juice and thus the treatment can be continued for several weeks at a time.

Camomile bath

Make a strong decoction in 2 pints of water and add to bath water. (See next chapter, p. 222.)

Cottage (curd) cheese

Warm up some sour milk to about 160°F. (70°C.)—not more—and drain off the whey through a cloth or bag. The firm mass which remains is the cheese. If it is hard and dry, it can be beaten up with a little fresh sour milk just before serving with the rawkost meal, or a little sweet milk for the cereal meal.

Another method: mix the sour milk with hot sweet milk in the proportion 3 to 1 and let the mixture stand 4 or 5 hours. Then strain off the whey as before.

Decoction for gastric ulcers

Soak 3 tablespoonfuls of whole linseed and 6 tablespoonfuls of wheat bran overnight in 3 pints of hot water. In the morning boil for 20 to 30 minutes until thick and slimy, from time to time thinning it down with a little water. Wash and cut into slices 1 lb. of raw potatoes, *with* the skins, and boil for about 20 minutes in 3 pints of water. This may also be diluted if it gets too thick. Strain both decoctions through a sieve and mix together while still hot and stand to cool. Care must be taken not to let it go sour.

During the first ten days of fasting, gastric-ulcer patients have 7 ozs. (1 teacup) of this decoction every two hours. If possible they should have, at the same time, half a cup of raw carrot juice added to the decoction, making the quantity up to a cup and a half. If the patient is at first unable to tolerate this quantity of raw carrot juice, it should be given 1 tablespoonful at a time, increasing the decoction so that the whole quantity taken each time is always 1½ cups. The drink should be taken seven times during the day from the time of waking.

The enema

Two forms of this treatment are prescribed: 1, the large, double enema, consisting of a preliminary injection of a pint of lukewarm water, immediately expelled and followed by a second, consisting of, 2 pints; 2, the small enema, consisting of 1 pint of cool (not cold) water.

This treatment is recommended as an aid to the elimination of toxins and waste matter during the change-over to the reformed diet, or during a fast and certain specified treatments. The chief aim of all bowel-cleansing treatments is, however, to encourage the bowel to function *naturally,* and it is important not to continue too long with daily or twice-daily enemas of the larger quantity which, unless otherwise stated, should never be taken for longer periods than one month. The small, cool enemas of only 1 pint may be continued as long as needed, as they have no relaxing effect. Used after a main meal, preferably the evening meal, when peristalsis (the muscular contractions of the bowel for propelling the fecal matter toward the exit) is normally active, the small enema is an excellent means of promoting regular bowel movements. Diminishing quantities will be needed until the bowel acts without assistance.

"Excelsior"—the morning drink

Potatoes in jackets, carrots, celery or celeriac, and any other root vegetables or left-over salads may be used. Clean thoroughly and boil for about half an hour in plenty of water—without salt, of course. Strain off the liquid and, in the evening, add to it 2 level tablespoonfuls of bran, 2 tablespoonfuls of whole linseed for each person, and allow to stand over night. On waking in the morning, warm up a pint of this drink for each person. If a still more concentrated decoction is desired, cut up the vegetables before cooking them. Stir when serving and while drinking so as to get all the bran and linseed.

Fasting on raw juices

During a fast the patient should drink daily 2 to 2½ quarts —never less, except in cases of severe heart or kidney disease, when the patient should have 1 to 1½ quarts daily. These patients may gradually increase the daily amount of fluid as their condition improves. It is important to drink slowly and mix the drink with the saliva.

Daily program for fasting

On waking: I pint of potato water or vegetable broth.

Breakfast, lunch, and dinner: up to a pint of juices of raw root or green vegetables. For *green* vegetables ⅓ juice to ⅔ potato water or vegetable broth. For *root* vegetables the proportion is reversed, i.e., ⅔ juice to ⅓ potato water or vegetable broth. After this, more of the broth if desired.

Midmorning and afternoon: a suitable herb tea (up to ¾ pint). Patients with heart or kidney troubles may very gradually increase the quantity of fluids.

Breaking the fast

First days

Breakfast: sour milk only, eaten very slowly.

Midmorning: herb tea.

Lunch: potatoes in jackets, boiled without salt, peeled and mashed with the fork. Sour milk.

Afternoon: herb tea.

Dinner: the same as lunch. Possibly a little slightly sweetened cranberry jam.

N.B. No *raw* juices in the morning or between meals; only potato water, "Excelsior," or herb teas.

After a fast of five days the patient may carefully begin to take normal diet on the *second day.*

After a fast of seven days the reversion may begin on the *third day* and

After a ten-day fast on the *fourth* day,
After a two-week fast on the *fifth* day,
After a three-week fast on the *sixth* day,
After a four-week fast on the *seventh* day.

Enemas

During the intervals between fasts, small, cool enemas of one pint should be taken—only when necessary—after dinner.

The limited diet

On waking: potato water or "Excelsior" (1 pint).

Breakfast: fruit, with a cup of herb or rose-hip tea. For excessively acid patients: 4/5 to 1 pint of raw vegetable juices (root vegetables diluted with 1/3 of this quantity of potato water or vegetable broth; green vegetables with 2/3).

Lunch and dinner: a small portion of sour milk; one large, or two small potatoes; plenty of *rawkost*

(salads). A little raw juice. At first no bread except "rheumatic bread"; later, one slice of wholemeal or crisp bread per day. No butter, only some cold pressed oil. No cheese except homemade curd (cottage) cheese.

Midmorning and afternoon: herb teas.

Highly alkaline diet

This is given in detail at the end of the chapter on rheumatic diseases. Based on the elimination of acid-forming foods, it is beneficial in all cases where overacidity is the cause—or one of the causes—of the trouble.

Avoidance of all fruit (except sweet, dried fruits), cereals, and strongly flavored roots, such as onions, garlic, and horseradish, is the chief feature of this diet. Two vegetable-and-salad meals are taken instead of one vegetable and one cereal meal per day. Rheumatic bread takes the place of wholemeal bread and potato porridge for breakfast and forms an alkaline complement to the sour milk.

Warm soda baths

In chronic cases of rheumatism warm soda baths followed by perspiring in bed are a very useful form of treatment. Great caution must be observed if the patient has a weak heart, and in acute cases no baths must be given until the acute stage is over and the temperature is normal.

Two pounds of washing soda are used for a bath. Commencing at a temperature of 99°F., the patient lies in the bath for 15 minutes, during which hot water is added until, if the patient's heart can stand it, the temperature has reached 104°F. Perspiration should begin in the bath and then continue in bed for about half an hour. After perspiring, the patient should be sponged with tepid water and then lie in bed for at least two hours. It is best not to leave the patient alone while perspiring, and the pulse should be checked from time to time.

Kruska

The best kruska is made from the four grains oatmeal, barley, wheat, and rye, ground at home just before cooking. This preserves the vitamins and auxones which are destroyed soon after grinding through exposure to the air. A hand mill or coffee mill, adjustable for coarser and finer grinding, should be used. To make one portion of kruska:

1	tablespoonful	whole	wheat
1	"	"	rye
1	"	"	barley
1	"	"	oats
1	"	"	wheat bran
1-2	"	raisins (with seeds when possible)	

Grind the grains very coarse and mix in two cups of boiling water. Boil rapidly for 5 minutes, not more, pour into a pre-heated thermos jug, or, if that is not available put the covered pan into a "hay box" (easily made of any large box or carton, packed tightly with newspaper all around the pan, and covered with a cushion). Leave to "draw" for *at least* half an hour, but preferably two hours or longer. It should still be steaming hot when taken up. Eat with milk and eventually stewed apple or dates. The only permissible addition to this meal, if desired, is wholemeal bread, butter and cottage or whey cheese.

If the four grains are not available, a very good kruska is made from *coarse* oatmeal ("pinhead" or coarser), bran and raisins, using 1 measure of oatmeal, 2 of bran, and 5 of water. Proceed as before. A very good kruska is also made of buckwheat, the only cereal which is basic; very rich in protein, easy to digest.

Molino

Two tablespoonfuls whole linseed, two tablespoonfuls wheat bran, one tablespoonful coarsely ground wheat flour, two or three cut-up figs, and a handful of raisins are cooked five minutes in a cup of water. The porridge is served immediately with sweet milk and possibly with a fruit compote or dried fruit, e.g., dates.

Onion poultice

Lay finely chopped red or yellow onion in a gauze bag, or bandage, on the part to be treated, or, if this causes too much pain, close to the sore. Fasten the poultice with adhesive tape or a gauze bandage. More closely woven fabric than surgical gauze should not be used. The poultice should be changed every four hours during the daytime and renewed during the night if the patient wakes up.

Potato porridge

Grate well-scrubbed potatoes (skins and all) over a pan of boiling water. Boil, stirring until the porridge thickens, and remove from heat. Some of the potato will be only half cooked, which is intentional. This can be served with either sweet or sour milk and is a good breakfast dish with dried fruit.

Raw vegetable juices

These can be made in several ways, the easiest being to use one of the various electric juice extractors. There are also good hand-operated juicers. The vegetables may even be run through a grinder or grated fine on a grater and then wrung out in a cloth. Careful note should be taken of instructions as to quantity and dilution of juices for acute conditions.

Rice kruska

Only unpolished "brown" rice should be used. This contains the valuable husk and the germ. The difference between polished and unpolished rice is about the same as between wholewheat bread and white bread.

Rice should be scalded once or twice before cooking.

Rice kruska is more easily digested than the more commonly used four-grain type. People who suffer from intestinal catarrh, for instance, find they can tolerate rice kruska better than other kinds.

Method: Use 3 tablespoonfuls of rice to ½ quart of water. Add dried fruit (prunes and figs, whole or cut into pieces; best if they have been soaked for a while). Boil the rice with the fruit 15-30 minutes. After cooking, put into a preheated thermos jug or hay box (see kruska recipe earlier in this chapter). Serve with fresh milk.

Sauerkraut *

To make a large supply for a family:
One bushel of white cabbage; two ounces of juniper berries.

The sauerkraut is made in a large earthenware crock, glazed inside. You will also require a lid, a heavy weight, and a clean towel.

First thoroughly clean and rinse the container, the lid, and other accessories required. Wash the cabbage leaves and cut them in thin shreds. Lay the first layer at the bottom of the crock and crush until the juice runs out and a froth is formed. Sprinkle a few juniper berries and put in the second layer, repeating the process until the container is nearly full. Lay a few large cabbage leaves on top and cover with a clean towel, newly washed and boiled. Finally, cover the whole with a few cabbage leaves with ventilation holes in them. Put the lid on and weight it down with a newly washed heavy stone, which will press

* See Glossary.

down the layers. The juice of the cabbage should cover all the layers.

Place the crock in a warm room so that fermentation starts as quickly as possible. Cover the crock with a clean cloth to protect from dust.

After a few days, and then every two or three days, remove all the scum. Each time, wash the cloth, the lid, and the stone in hot water. When the scum no longer rises, the process of fermentation is finished and the crock can be put in a cool place.

The sauerkraut will be ready to eat in four weeks at the latest. Each time the crock is opened to take out the cabbage, the lid, the towel, and the stone must be washed in hot water. The inner rim and walls of the crock must be kept very clean—this is the only way to preserve the fresh, flavor of the cabbage.

Sourdough *

This method of leavening bread was customary for hundreds of years. It consists in putting aside a lump of dough when baking and keeping it to leaven the next batch.

Sour milk—Filbunke

In Sweden, at least four kinds of sour milk are commonly used, including "long milk" * and yogurt. The simplest, however, is the homemade variety known as *filbunke*.* This is prepared as follows:

* See page 18.

Take the cream from the top of a milk bottle and stand in a warm place until thick. Use this as a culture; put 1-1½ tablespoons of it into a bowl (for one portion), smearing the sides, and add half a pint of milk to each bowl (in cold weather warm the milk slightly—up to 90°F.). Stir well till smooth, cover and stand in a warm (not hot) place until set. When serving, reserve a spoonful or two as culture for each new portion. Milk should be *unpasteurized* whenever possible. Serve in the original bowls, undisturbed. It should set after about 24 hours—perhaps longer in winter. At the table, top the bowl with bran, linseed, and milk sugar and eat with fresh fruit if in normal health.

*Long Milk.** For this a special culture is required.

Sprouted soya beans

Same as for wheat.

Sprouted wheat

Soak the wheat grains in water at room temperature overnight. In the morning, spread out thinly on a dish or on a sheet of brown paper. Do this for three days. To prevent the grains from going sour, they must be rinsed under running water three times a day. A warm room, out of the

* See glossary.

draft, is the best place to sprout the grains. When the sprouts are ⅛ inch long, they are ready to use. In winter they often take four days to sprout. One or two tablespoonfuls daily is the normal quantity per person.

Vegetable broth

As for "Excelsior" before adding linseed and bran.

Yogurt

The effectiveness of yogurt lies in the particular bacteria used in its preparation. The milk is heated to a temperature sufficiently high to destroy other bacteria already present in the milk. Then it is inoculated with the desired bacteria and kept at the temperature best suited to their growth. When the bacteria have reached the desired concentration, the yogurt is refrigerated.

Mrs. Waerland prefers home-soured milk to yogurt. But since many people are unwilling or have little time to bother with making it, she permits good-quality commercial yogurt in its place.

Yogurt and other kinds of sour milk combine well with fresh and dried fruits and raw vegetables and aid in their digestion. Sour milk should not be eaten with carbohydrate foods when these consitute the main part of the meal. Thus, in the regular Waerland diet, sour milk is eaten with fruit for breakfast and with the *rawkost* meal but not with the cereal meal.

24 / *Nature's rich dispensary: herbs*

Knowledge of the healing properties of herbs and trees is very old. In ancient Greece the effect of medicinal herbs on ailments was already known, and the physicians of that day used natural methods in treating disease.

In the Middle Ages the monks cultivated medicinal plants in the gardens of their monasteries and used them to heal the sick. The Herbals of those days contain a wealth of knowledge in this field. "Wise women" and "wizards" inherited this art from the monks and often achieved wonderful results with their "simples."

Anyone who makes a deep study of nature's sources of healing cannot fail to be filled with reverence for the Creator who gave such wonderful properties to our most humble plants and ordinary trees, all so ingeniously adapted to the complicated workings of the body that they never do it any harm when used with discrimination.

How different are the synthetic remedies which, although they suppress the symptoms of disease, leave the source of it untouched, often even damaging vital organs and upsetting the functions of the body. Innumerable examples could be given of this, not least the findings of present-day research concerning the entirely wrong composition of our remedies for sleeplessness and their harmful effect on the nervous system.

As the art of medicine becomes more enlightened, there will be a reversion to the infinitely rich store offered us in nature's "dispensary." This new biological age has already entered upon fresh trends in science and invention, and we shall come closer to nature than in the mechanical era.

Juniper

The berries of this often despised bush, gathered in the autumn and dried in the sun, are an ancient remedy for many different ailments. They are rich in volatile oils which increase the flow of blood to the mucous membrane and regulate the activity of the digestive glands and the muscles of the stomach and intestines. This makes the berries very useful in affections of the mucous membranes of the stomach and bowels, and in disturbances in the functioning of the kidneys, liver, and gall resulting from pathological changes in the mucous membranes of the digestive tract. They are also beneficial for infectious lung diseases. The volatile oils are fatal to bacteria and, being soluble in fats, are able to penetrate into the body of the bacteria. Their action on the tissues of the lungs and bronchial tubes is particularly helpful on this account, as they lessen the further excretion of the glands while, at the same time, stimulating the action of the mucous membrane whereby the elimination of the existing excretion is assisted. Nevertheless, in cases of ordinary bronchial catarrh, juniper berries should not be used, as it is important not to inhibit the excretion of mucus, which in this case is part of a natural cleansing process.

While some of the volatile oils are eliminated via the lungs, most of them are dealt with by the kidneys, the excretion of urine being thereby increased. In cases of dropsy, edema, and swollen limbs, and for rheumatism and gout, juniper berries are beneficial but may *not* be used where there is inflammation of the kidneys.

Metabolism is stimulated by juniper berries, and they relieve the pains of menstruation, if there is cramp, by increasing the flow of blood.

Method of using juniper

A juniper cure is carried out in this way: on the first day five berries are taken, on the second day six, the third day seven, and so on until one has reached fifteen berries. Then one less berry is taken each day until down to five again. If this cure is repeated four or five times the most unhealthy blood can be purified.

If juniper berries are to be used as a *diuretic,* they should be made into a tea: 1 tablespoonful of crushed berries boiled in 2 cupfuls of water, taken in sips during the course of the day.

Compresses made with a decoction of juniper can be used to *relieve the pain of arthritis.* For this, take 1 lb. of juniper twigs and pour over them 6 quarts of hot water. Next morning boil for 20 minutes to half an hour. Strain and use the liquid for compresses. Put on the affected part as hot as possible.

Willow Bark

This has been used medicinally for two thousand years. It was still in use only a hundred years ago as a remedy for *rheumatism* and for *fever*.

Willow bark contains the substance *salizin*, which the body converts into salicylic acid to reduce fever and alleviate pain. Synthetic preparations of salicylic acid, injurious to the mucous membranes of the stomach and intestines, are now used instead of this harmless, natural substance.

Tea made from willow bark induces gentle perspiration: 15 grams (½ oz.) of bark infused in three cups of boiling water. Allow to stand and draw overnight, then boil for five minutes. Drink during the course of the day. Tea can also be made from powdered bark without boiling. For this, take 1 or 2 teaspoonfuls of powdered bark to 2 cups of boiling water. Allow to draw for 8 hours. The tea is best taken after meals. In cases of rheumatism and arthritis, equal amounts of willow bark and birch leaves can be mixed, using one or two teaspoonfuls of the mixture to each cup of water, prepared in the same way. Three cups of this should be taken daily.

During the great shortage of drugs in Germany, in and following the second world war, doctors made clinical experiments with willow bark and got excellent results in acute and chronic cases of muscular rheumatism and arthritis, neuralgia, migraine, lumbago, and influenza. Seventy per cent of all cases treated were completely restored within a short time, which goes to show that better results may be obtained with natural herbal drugs than with synthetic preparations.

The apple

This is the king of fruits. We have always known that the apple was a wholesome fruit, rich in vitamins, but it is only recently that science has discovered its unique medicinal value. In 1919 a German physician, Dr. Heisler, was called to see a patient who had been suffering for four weeks from acute intestinal catarrh and was exhausted and emaciated. None of the remedies tried had done any good. Dr. Heisler had heard of a man who had cured himself very quickly of long-standing and very severe intestinal catarrh by a diet of grated raw apples, and he decided to try an experiment. To his great astonishment, the patient recovered within a few days. Another German physician, Kutroff who had a large hospital near the western front, cured the most severe cases of dysentery with apples. He gave his patients $1\frac{1}{2}$ kilos (about $3\frac{1}{3}$ pounds) of grated raw apples daily. He also used whole apples, which had to be very well chewed. Most of the cases were cured within two days and improved noticeably in one day. Similar apple cures have since then been practiced in a great many hospitals.

Method: 1 to $1\frac{1}{2}$ kg. (2 to $3\frac{1}{3}$ lbs.) of unpeeled apples. Remove the cores and grate on a glass grater. This quantity should be taken in 8 portions during the course of the day. It is important that the patient take *no medicine of any kind* during the apple cure.

The apples act as a sponge in the intestine, absorbing liquid and toxic matter which is then quickly expelled. It is the content of volatile substances—tannic acid, fruit acids, and minerals—which effects the rapid cure. Excellent results have been achieved with this treatment in cases of gastric and intestinal catarrh, paratyphoid, and dysentery.

A well-known children's physician, Dr. Moro, had some splendid results with children suffering from diarrhea and dysentery. After two days on apples only, he gradually changed the diet back to ordinary food but continued for some time with decreasing portions of apple.

In the peel of the apple there is a substance, pectin, which has the quality of causing blood to congeal. This is now largely used in treating cases of excessive bleeding.

The apple is also excellent for treating diseases affecting metabolism. Even with cooked apples, doctors have had very good results in treating dropsy, also diseases of the heart and blood vessels. These patients had about 3 pounds of stewed apples slightly sweetened, with no other food, on three days in the week.

Apples are particularly useful for treating *anemia,* being rich in iron, arsenic, and phosphorous. They are also good for intellectual workers.

Nerve specialists in Germany use apple juice as an effective remedy in nervous cases and have established that they have a calming and relaxing effect.

Rose hips

Most people know that rose hips are an excellent source of vitamin C. But not everyone knows that they are almost our *best* source of this vitamin. According to the findings of reliable research, rose hips contain five times as much vitamin C as oranges and lemons. 100 grams (3½ oz.) of rose hips contain as much as 200 milligrams (1/140 oz.) of vitamin C. Boiling reduces the vitamin content by half, but, even then, the rose hips exceed the citrus fruits in vitamin content. Therefore, in rose-hip tea, rose-hip soup (used for dessert in Sweden), and rose-hip jam we are able to cover our needs for vitamin C without resorting to the fruits from the South.

The oak

In ancient times the oak was a sacred tree.

The bark of the oak is rich in *tannin,* which has astringent and blood-checking qualities known ever since the first century A.D. Naturopaths now use the bark of the oak as a remedy both internally and externally. For blood spitting, bronchial catarrh, chronic gastric catarrh, diarrhea, and hemorrhoids, a useful *decoction can be made as follows:*

> 15 grams (½ oz.) of powdered oak boiled for ten minutes in ½ liter (1 pt.) of water. This can be sweetened with honey.

For weakness of the urinary bladder, another decoction is made thus: 10 grams (⅓ oz.) powdered oak bark and a few crushed juniper berries boiled for five minutes in ¼ liter (½ pt.) of milk. 2 to 3 tablespoonfuls to be taken morning and evening with a little honey.

Externally, the decoction of oak is used as a gargle for a sore throat and swollen tonsils, and it can very well be used as a fomentation for chilblains, boils, and skin eruptions; it is also useful for perspiration of the feet with unpleasant odor. *To make a decoction for external use:*

30 gr. (1 oz.) powdered oak bark boiled in 1½ liters (3 pts.) of water until only two pints remain (20 to 30 minutes).

As a douche for personal hygiene for women, a decoction of oak bark can be used to heal irritated membranes. For this, boil 1 part of bark for 15 minutes in 15 parts of water. A slightly weaker decoction is useful for bed sores.

Acorns are used by country people for cancer and leucorrhea and sore membranes. The following decoction is used: the acorns are shelled and cut in thin slices or grated (finely grated acorns can be bought at a druggist's). One tablespoonful is put on in 1 liter (1 qt.) of cold water and boiled for five minutes. Drink during the day.

The birch

This beautiful northern tree, with its fair white trunk, admired and sung by poets, a symbol of spring and romance when putting forth its tender green leaves, contains also many healing properties both in leaves and in sap. As long ago as the thirteenth century, birch-leaf tea was used for fevers and diseases of the stomach and chest. And as early as the sixteenth century the sweet sap of the birch was used in the spring just as in the present day. To get the sap, a hole is bored in the trunk and a container hung below it to catch the liquid. This is excellent as a blood purifier.

Birch-leaf tea is used for rheumatic diseases, skin eruptions, inflammation of the bladder, and anemia. *To prepare:* take two tablespoonfuls of dried birch leaves, cut them fine, and pour over them two cupfuls of boiling water. Allow to draw for a while, then boil up quickly. Allow to stand for two hours, then strain and allow to cool. Drink cold, morning, midday, and evening.

An excellent tea for purifying the blood is made from 2 parts of birch leaves, 1 part of stinging nettles, 1 part of elder flowers, and 1 part of sloe flowers (blackthorn).* For every cup of tea, use 1 tablespoonful of the mixture which is infused in boiling water. Allow to draw. Three cups of this should be taken daily for a month.

In the thirteenth century, fomentations of birch leaves were used for rheumatism. The patient was swathed in blankets over the fomentations, which induced copious perspiration: birch leaves are highly diaphoretic, or sweat-producing.

Dr. Winternitz, the well-known professor, has shown that birch-leaf tea is such a powerful diuretic that the quantity of urine is often increased by eight times. But the remarkable thing is that this extra functioning of the kidneys is not accompanied by the slightest irritation. He also

* *blackthorn: Prunus spinosa,* whose fruit is used to flavor drinks. The American *blackthorn* (*Crataegus tomentosa*) is an entirely different tree.

established that the excretion of albumin in the urine was lessened. He therefore recommends birch-leaf tea as an excellent remedy for disorders of the urinary tract.

In France, Dr. Huchard had very good results with birch-leaf tea in treating gout. Dr. Jännicke also used the tea successfully for kidney stones. He found that all adverse symptoms disappeared after a period of treatment and that the stones were passed at first in pieces the size of a pea and later as sand.

Preparation: 1 teaspoonful of dried, fine-cut birch leaves to each cup of water. Infuse in boiling water and allow to draw. One cup to be taken in the morning on an empty stomach and another at about five in the afternoon. The patient does this for at least a month in conjunction with the diet for kidney and gallstone troubles described in this book.

Professor Bohn used birch-leaf tea made of fresh young leaves for rheumatism, gout, and kidney disease. Birch-leaf tea drives the uric acid out of the body. The many versatile uses and the efficacy of birch leaves are due to the potassium salts they contain, and also to the presence of *saponin* substances, which are diaphoretic.

Birch tar has been used for hundreds of years for treating skin diseases. It is obtainable at drugstores.

Pine and spruce

These also have medicinal qualities. Tender shoots, gathered in the spring and made into a decoction, either fresh or dried, are good for coughs and cystitis.

Preparation: 15 grams (½ oz.) boiled for 10 minutes in ½ liter (1 pt.) of water.

Spruce cones produce excellent medicine for colds, hoarseness, and coughs. The cones should be gathered in September and boiled in a large amount of water for five hours. The liquid is then strained and boiled again with syrup until thick. It is then bottled, corked, and sealed with resin.

Pine-needles baths are excellent for colds, rheumatism, sciatica, conditions of cramp, overstrain, sleeplessness, and neuralgia. The first bath should last ten minutes; subsequent baths half an hour. Both spruce and pine needles induce increased flow of blood to both surface and deep-seated disease.

A decoction for baths can be made at home by soaking spruce or pine twigs in boiling water overnight and boiling it up the next day for half an hour. But very large vessels are required for this, as 1 to 1½ kilograms (2 to 3 lbs.) of twigs are needed for each bath.

Elder

This tree was brought to the northern countries centuries ago from Central Europe. It was regarded as a sacred tree, the home of the goddess Freja, the defender against all evil. Before the coming of Christianity, no one might pass an elder bush without a salutation and, as a token of reverence, either taking off the hat or bowing the head. It was not long before people discovered that in the elder they could find a cure for many ills. Long before the monks brought the knowledge of herbal remedies to the North, our heathen forefathers had planted the elder beside every dwelling so as to have a household dispensary close at hand. The *root* supplied a laxative, the *bark* was laid on inflamed places, the *leaves* were used for burns, the *berries* as a diuretic, also the *flowers,* but these were also used for wounds.

Elder flowers contain a volatile oil which encourages perspiration. For *fevers* a tea is made from the flowers, one to two cups to be taken at bedtime as warm as possible, and once or twice during the day. *To make elderflower tea* use 1-2 tablespoonfuls of the flowers and infuse in 1 pt. of boiling water, allowing it to draw for ten minutes. A little lemon juice and honey may be added.

Elder flowers also contain a sex hormone and are therefore beneficial at the climacteric. The berries are rich in vitamin C. *A delicious puree* can be made from elderberries: gently boil ripe berries in a little water for a little while, stirring all the time. Press the juice through a cloth. To every quart of juice add half a pound of sugar, or less if the sharp flavor is liked. Boil, stirring all the time, until the juice and sugar form a thin puree. Put into jars and cover.

Lime or linden (Tilia)

The medicinal properties of the lime are well known, especially in cases of influenza and colds. *Lime-flower tea* encourages perspiration (diaphoretic). *An excellent blend,* if the lime flower alone is not desirable, is 10 grams (⅓ oz.) of lime flower, 20 grams (⅔ oz.) of wild pansy ("heartsease"), 10 grams (⅓ oz.) of camomile flowers, and 10 grams (⅓ oz.) of elder flowers. To each cup of boiling water use one tablespoonful of the blend and allow to draw. Sweeten with honey. This tea is very beneficial and pleasant to the taste.

The linden tree has long been affectionately associated with the poetry and romance of home life in northern Europe and was given a place of honor beside every cottage and farmhouse as the Guardian Tree, with which the life of the family was intimately connected. Lime-flower tea, *tilleul,* is a popular beverage in France.

Camomile (Anthemis nobilis)

This is also a well-known medicinal plant, widely used. There is another plant, very similar to camomile, but having none of its beneficial qualities: the dog's fennel, or mayweed (*Anthemis cotula*). True camomile is distinguishable from this by its sweet, spicy perfume and bitter taste; it is smaller than the dog fennel, and the receptacle, or center, is more semiglobular in shape.

Ever since the days of Disocorides, the Greek physician, camomile has been used to relieve the pains of childbirth and menstruation. This is because of its relaxing effect on cramped conditions and its sedative, healing qualities.

Camomile Tea: 1 teaspoonful to 1 tablespoonful of flowers to half a pint of water. Infuse in boiling water and allow to draw for 10 minutes. *For external use:* 1 to 5 tablespoonfuls of flowers to 2 pints of boiling water.

Camomile is a useful *disinfectant* and makes a good gargle for sore throat or as a mouth wash for blisters or ulcers. It is useful for washing sores and has a healing action when used as an enema for intestinal catarrh, fistulas, or sores in the rectum. For inflamed eyes, use as an eye bath. For drawing out matter, as in the case of *boils,* fill a small muslin bag with the flowers, warm it, and place on the affected part.

The effective constituents of camomile are mainly a volatile oil and a glucoside, and it is, as we have seen, an internal and external remedy of great value.

As camomile relaxes cramp, it can also be used for pain in passing water. *Dr. Aschner* uses it for most children's ailments, especially for diarrhea and during teething, when it is useful in many ways.

Dr. Steinmetz has established that camomile tea can increase the flow of bile by 100%.

Professor Delondre recommends a cup of camomile tea as an excellent remedy for sleeplessness.

Camomile poultices, or compresses, are beneficial for rashes and irritations of the skin, such as eczema.

A very effective *decoction for arresting diarrhea* is prepared thus: 50 grams (1⅔ oz.) of camomile, 15 grams (½ oz.) of dried blueberries, 10 grams (⅓ oz.) of powdered oak bark. Mix together and use 1 tablespoonful to half a pint of water. Boil for a few minutes.

For *sleeplessness* an excellent tea is a blend of equal parts of hops, salvia, and camomile, just brought to the boil.

Hawthorn

An effective remedy for heart troubles is to be found in this shrub. In the *hawthorn* there has been discovered considerable quantities of aluminum, potassium, sodium, calcium, and phosphorus, besides tannin and saponin substances. It has been scientifically established that the flowers and fruit are a nonpoisonous remedy for heart diseases and disturbances of the blood-vessel system. They also relieve cramp and can be used for inhibited functioning of the kidneys. Some doctors even think that for local heart disturbances, especially angina pectoris, the hawthorn is superior to digitalis. In the nineteenth century, doctors in England and France began to use an essence of hawthorn for angina pectoris, enlarged heart, and weakness of the heart, also for nervous disturbances of the heart and intestines.

Hawthorn drops—crataegus—can be obtained from homeopathic druggists. When this is taken in a dose of *5 drops on an empty stomach*, it is most effective. But a home-brewed tea can be made of the flowers and fruit (fresh or dried). Equal parts of each are taken and 1 tablespoonful used to 1 cup of boiling water. Allow to draw, and drink in small doses during the day.

Fern

Both root and leaves of this highly radioactive plant have their uses. The roots should be gathered in dry weather in the late autumn, branch roots, soil, and the leafy fronds removed, and the main roots, with the two-inch-long stems of the fronds, put to dry in an airy place without washing, peeling, or cutting. Only healthy roots should be used. Roots gathered in the summer are worthless.

Medicinal ferns and bracken are much alike. The best way of recognizing the medicinal fern is to look at the stalk: cut off a frond close to the ground, and if the cut section is in the form of a rounded triangle, it is the right plant. The section of the bracken stalk is flat and two-sided. Only fresh green leaves should be harvested.

Ferns were used as early as the third century A.D. as a remedy for tapeworms and are used to this day by both orthodox and naturopathic doctors for the same purpose. This is the most effective remedy there is, and it is known to Indians and Negro races.

Naturopaths use the medicinal fern for a number of ailments, especially *rheumatism. For use in the bath,* 1 kilogram (2⅕ lbs.) of fern root, finely cut, should be boiled in 6 liters (6⅓ quarts) of water for one hour. The bath should be quite warm.

For goitre, a decoction of medicinal fern is very good. Cut a large root into small pieces and boil in 3 liters (3 qts.) of vinegar. Strain, allow to cool, and rub in.

Arthritic patients benefit from sleeping on fern fronds. Wearing fern fronds in the shoes and taking a hot footbath with a decoction of fern in it at night helps one to sleep well. But care must be taken to gather the plant in dry weather only. For *muscular rheumatism,* fine-cut fern root in a small linen bag placed on the painful spot will help. The pain will be relieved after only a couple of hours, because the fern root stimulates the circulation of the blood in the affected muscles and the tension is relieved. Best of all, the improvement is lasting.

Tincture of fern is one of the best remedies for rheumatism. Take young, fresh fronds, cut up fine, and place in a glass or jar and cover with brandy. Cover the jar with parchment paper and stand in the sun or other warm place for a week. Pour off the spirit, and it will be found to have absorbed all the curative properties of the fern. This tincture will keep for years and can be applied to the painful places, not only in rheumatism but for inflammation, swellings, bruises, and blows.

Dried fern fronds which have been picked when young and fresh retain the same wonderful radioactive properties as the fresh fronds for at least a year.

Common spotted fern (Polypodium vulgare)

The root of this fern is good for constipation, asthma, and hoarseness. For diseases of the *throat and chest:* pour half a liter (1 pint) of boiling water on 8 to 16 grams (2/7 to 4/7 ozs.) of the root and boil it. *For stomach and intestinal troubles:* 40 to 50 grams to 1 liter (1⅓ to 1¾ ozs. to 1 quart) of water; boil for 20 minutes and take two cups daily.

Professor Volmar found that the decoction of spotted fern would promote a painless bowel movement after ten hours and also increase the activity of the gall. *For constipation* make the following decoction: boil 20 grams (¾ oz.) of the root in ¾ liter (¾ quart), then add 10 grams (⅓ oz.) of licorice and 5 grams (⅙ oz.) of angelica root to the boiling liquid. Remove from heat and allow to stand undisturbed for twelve hours. Sweeten with honey and drink in the morning on an empty stomach.

Yarrow (Achillea millefolium)

Both flowers and leaves can be used. The flowers can be gathered all summer in dry weather, but the leaves should preferably be picked before the flowering.

In ancient Greece this herb was used for wounds and sores, and it is not very long since soldiers used to carry it in their knapsacks. Even in the ninth century an ointment was made in Iceland from the finely-chopped leaves and used for sores and rashes. In England it is still used as a beauty preparation. If for some time the face is washed in yarrow tea, the skin will become firm and lines and wrinkles be prevented.

Preparation: Tea from the flowers—1 tablespoonful of flowers to 1 cup of boiling water. For *chronic bronchial catarrh:* 3 cups per day. *Tea from the leaves:* 20 grams (⅔ oz.) to 2 cups of boiling water. For *kidney* and *bladder* troubles, *kidney stone,* and *menstrual* trouble, the tea should be taken in sips during the course of the day. This tea is also good for *bedwetting.* A strong decoction of the whole herb is used for treating sores and suppurations. Early scientific medicine used yarrow for bleeding piles, gastric and intestinal catarrh, and chronic enlargement of the liver.

Tea made from flowers and leaves is highly stimulating to the metabolism. It also stimulates the circulation and is therefore good for people who have sensations of numbness in hands and feet. As it relieves cramp, it is beneficial for *angina pectoris.* The fresh juice, used as a lotion, is good for varicose veins.

Lady's Mantle (Alchemilla vulgaris)

Lady's Mantle is mentioned in the herbals of the thirteenth century as an excellent healer for sores and as a remedy for epilepsy. For the latter, the juice should be drunk in the morning on an empty stomach. *Preparation for sores:* use the whole plant, pouring 1 liter (1 quart) of boiling water over 30 grams (1 oz.) of the herb. Dip a compress in the tea and lay upon the sore. Lady's Mantle is also used *internally* to *stimulate metabolism.* A strong decoction—60 grams to 1 liter (2 ozs. to 1 qt.)—of water is used for *excessive menstrual flow* and *intestinal catarrh.* Cut up the herb fine and use 3 teaspoonfuls to 300 grams ($\frac{3}{10}$ quart) of water, boiling for a minute or two. Allow to draw, and drink one to two cups daily. Lady's Mantle is rich in tannin and also contains saponin. If it is blended with equal parts of cowslip, it makes a very fine tea, excelling all others in aroma and flavor.

Heather

This is an ancient remedy. A decoction of heather—10 grams ($\frac{1}{3}$ oz.) to a cup of water—can be used for a *cough* and stronger decoctions for *rheumatism* and *kidney stones.* Weak heather tea is an excellent soporific for children.

During the war, in Germany, the pillows of wounded soldiers were filled with heather and they were able to sleep in spite of their pains. Heather can only be used while flowering, when it should always be gathered. Only the tips of the branches, bearing the flowers, should be used.

Horsetail (Equisetum arvense)

This is the herb most used at Kiholm, Sweden, because, being a strong diuretic, it is excellent for rheumatism and kidney and bladder ailments. It is rich in silicic acid and belongs to the saponaceous plants. It should be gathered from June to September and—unlike most other medicinal herbs—should be dried *in the sun.* (All the others must be dried in the shade in an airy place.) There are several varieties of Horsetail (*Equisetum*) which are the relics of a group of plants which flourished in the Paleozoic Age, when they were of gigantic size.

Horsetail is an excellent remedy for *internal bleeding,* e.g., if the patient is coughing up or vomiting blood, and consequently in *tuberculosis. A decoction* is made for this —10 grams (⅓ oz.) to a cup. For *bladder trouble,* use a blend of horsetail, rose hips, and juniper—1 tablespoonful to a cup.

As an *external remedy,* this herb is used in the form of a decoction for *suppurating sores.* Use the liquid for cleaning the sore, then put some of the boiled herbs in a piece of gauze and lay it on the place. Well-known doctors have obtained excellent results by treating chronic *leg ulcers* in this way. For *catarrh of the bladder and the renal pelvis,* use 15 grams (½ oz.) of horsetail boiled in 1 liter (1 qt.) of water for half an hour. Drink half in the morning and half in the evening.

The content of silicic acid makes horsetail very good for lung troubles. The patient's appetite improves, fever and night sweating cease, and the bacillus content of the sputum decreases. The supply of minerals in the body is replenished. A *strengthening tonic* is made thus: boil 30 grams (1 oz.) of horsetail in 1 liter (1 qt.) of water for half an hour. Drink half a cup at intervals during the day.

Professor Hugo Schultz considers horsetail one of the best silicic drugs. This herb gives excellent results in the external treatment of *acute eczema* with baths and compresses.

Eyebright

This herb should be gathered—whole—in August and September. It is an excellent eye remedy for both external and internal use. *Decoction:* 1 tablespoonful of dried eyebright boiled for a few minutes in 300 grams (⅓ qt.) of water and strained. Use lukewarm for bathing inflamed eyes and for suppuration or mucous discharge of the conjunctivae and oversensitivity to light. *Internally,* a cupful of the same decoction taken in sips during the day. Eyebright is also good for the mucous membranes of the throat, lungs, and digestive tract.

Dandelion

The dandelion is, of all herbs, one of the richest in nutritional salts. It is a strong diuretic and blood purifier. The main roots should be gathered early in spring before the "rosette" of leaves has developed, or in October and November.

Arabian physicians in the early Middle Ages used the dandelion as an *eye remedy*. The Greek name for it (*taraxacum*) means "cures eye disease." The dandelion encourages the digestion and promotes menstruation, the high content of potassium stimulating the urinary organs while the bitter substances increase the activity of the glands secreting the digestive juices.

The percentage of nutritional salts in the dandelion is 1.9, consisting of potassium 38%, calcium 20%, sodium 11%, magnesium 9%, phosphorus 8%, silicium 7%, sulphur and chlorine 3%. The herb is rich in vitamin C, containing the bitter substances saponin and colocynthin, and is stimulating to all the glands of the body. The content of inulin, a carbohydrate allied to starch, in the root may be as much as 40%. It also contains levulin, which corresponds to the dextrine of starch.

Dried dandelion root is very valuable. When collected, the roots should be washed and the small rootlets can be wiped off with a cloth. The main roots should then be spread out to dry in an airy place out of the sun. The leaves, also, should be dried and can be used to make a tea for stimulating the appetite, as a diuretic and to increase the flow of bile. Fresh juice, made by wringing the chopped leaves in a cloth, is an excellent tonic.

Preparation to be used as a remedy for *promoting increased urine and bile:* 1 tablespoonful of the root boiled in ¾ liter (¾ qt.) of water. Drink 2 or 3 cups daily. *The leaves,* fresh or dry, can also be used for this and to stimulate the *appetite*. Two tablespoonfuls of dried leaves and root boiled for 10 minutes in 600 grams (21 ozs. = ⅔ quart) of water. Take two cups daily. Dandelion is also very good for *rheumatism.* Dandelion leaves are excellent for salads.

Coltsfoot (Tussilago farfara)

This is one of the oldest European *cough remedies.* Hippocrates called it *becchion,* which means "I drive out the cough." The flowers should be collected while freshly blooming, and the leaves in May and June. The leaves are not to be confused with those of the *Petasites officinalis,* which they resemble. These are kidney-shaped and covered with grayish hairs, whereas, the coltsfoot leaves are in the shape of a horseshoe with white hairs. The fresh leaves, crushed, are good for inflammations of the skin.

For hoarseness, coughs, and influenza, use a tea as follows: 5 to 10 grams (⅙ to ⅓ oz.) coltsfoot leaves infused in 1 cup of boiling water. Allow to draw for 10 minutes and strain. For *asthma:* 3 parts of coltsfoot, 3 parts sage, and 3 parts plantain. 10 grams (⅓ oz.) of this blend infused in half a liter (1 pint) of boiling water, strained after 15 minutes and sweetened with honey. One tablespoonful of this to be taken every hour.

The stinging nettle

This humble plant contains even more of the mineral salts than the dandelion. None of the wild herbs excels it in its wealth of organic salts and, of cultivated plants, only the gooseberry and the pea. It contains 2.3% of mineral salts, of which 32% is potassium, 29% calcium, 8% phosphorus, sulphur, and so on. On this account it has a great influence on the metabolism. The nettle is a good source of vitamin A, is rich in vitamin C, and also contains vitamin B. *Rheumatism and stone of the kidneys and bladder* are successfully treated with nettle juice and nettle tea. For the tea: boil 2 or 3 tablespoonfuls of fine-cut dried nettle leaves in half a liter (one pt.) of water for five minutes. Drink 1 or 2 cups daily. The *whole* of the nettle, but especially the seeds, is beneficial for all kinds of bleeding. *Best as raw juice.* Owing to its rich content of iron and chlorophyll, the nettle is as useful as spinach for enriching the blood.

Stewed nettles make a dainty dish: take some young nettles, well washed and shaken to remove the water; place in a pan with a lid, without any water but with a little butter. When tender, cut up in the pan.

The nutritional value of the nettle is twice that of the carrot. It contains, among other things, protein, fat, carbohydrate, and glucose. Nettles should be dried in an airy, shady place. They will dry in a day or two and should then be put into a bag with air holes in it.

Cold tea made from the dried leaves is an excellent mealtime *beverage*. *Infuse* 10 to 15 grams (⅓ to ½ oz.) of dried leaves in 1 liter (1 qt.) of boiling water and allow to draw before straining off the liquid. All the mineral salts are contained in this tea in large quantities.

The cabbage leaf

There are many variations of the cabbage, which is one of the few cultivated plants indigenous to Europe. In its wild state it has hard, sharp leaves, and only careful cultivation has produced the edible varieties. Cabbage not only is one of the most common and cheapest of foods but is also exceptional in its medicinal properties. It was a universal remedy even in ancient times, and for six hundred years the Romans used hardly any other healing agent. They used cabbage for both internal and external treatment, for poultices and compresses and treating sores, even as a remedy for the plague. For six hundred years the health of the Roman people was at a very high level, but with the spread of immorality and the lapse from good, wholesome ways, new and hitherto unknown diseases broke out and new remedies began to be used.

The honor of having rediscovered the wonderful, almost incomprehensible healing properties of the cabbage leaf must be given to Dr. Blanc, physician at the Hospice de Romans, Drôme. In a work published in 1881 he wrote: "Among remedies the cabbage plant should occupy the same position as that of bread among foods. The cabbage leaf is the poor man's doctor. It is a most effective remedy, with enormous possibilities."

Dr. Blanc describes many interesting cases which he cured with cabbage compresses. His first case was a badly ulcerated leg. The septic matter had to be drawn out before the healing process could begin. How was he to do this? All other methods had failed. Intuitively, Dr. Blanc had the idea of trying the cabbage leaf and, to his amazement, it succeeded. After only half a day of the treatment a thick, evil-smelling liquid began to discharge from the ulcer and the skin became softer and thinner. The dressings were changed twice a day, and soon the ulcer grew shallower and the surrounding tissues took on a lighter, more wholesome hue. Finally, a well-healed scar was all that remained of the long-standing, deeply infected ulcer.

Dr. Blanc repeated the experiment, with always the same result, in the treatment of protracted, infected sores. But how was the superiority of the cabbage leaf to all other remedies for inflamed sores to be explained? This was a problem to which he gave profound thought. He finally came to the conclusion that the cabbage leaf must have a special affinity with the septic matter which prevented the healing of the sores. This conclusion was supported by the strong secretion which invariably appeared when the cabbage treatment was used. It drew out the poisonous matter, thus cleansing the tissues so that they were able to heal. Dr. Blanc now found that he could prevent boils and ulcers by treating, in the early stages, spots and blisters which are the first indications of an unhealthy condition of the blood and tissues. In this way he cured all kinds of eruptions, even psoriasis and "scald-head" (scab) in babies. He also treated *headache, migraine, neuralgia,* and *rheumatism* with good results. It may sound like a fairy tale, but the fact that Dr. Blanc also had good results in treating *tumors* with cabbage leaves can only be attributed to their exceptional healing properties.

Encouraged by Dr. Blanc's wonderful experience, a number of other well-known doctors have tested the unique effects of the humble cabbage.

Dr. Blanc's book is full of examples of severe cases he cured with the cabbage treatment. Here are a few typical ones:

A boy was run over by a carriage. One of the wheels went over his leg. He was taken to the hospital and examined by three doctors, who all thought the leg would have to be amputated. The operation was put off till the next day, however. The same afternoon, someone thought of trying a cabbage compress. The boy was in great pain and very restless. The first compress was put on at five o'clock, and not long afterward he was calmer and the pain had lessened. He slept well all night until eight o'clock in the morning, when the doctors came and removed the cabbage compress, which was found to be soaked with bloody liquid. On washing the wound, it was found that the inflammation had subsided and the improvement was so great that an operation became unnecessary.

An old man had kidney trouble, catarrh of the bladder, stones in the urinary bladder, and cramp in the urethra.

Pain was severe and nothing did any good. Dr. Blanc ordered cabbage compresses over the abdomen and the kidneys. This treatment was begun on July 9, 1871. On the eleventh Dr. Blanc was informed that the discharge was so copious that it had saturated all the dressings and bedding. On the surface of the leaves which had been placed over the kidneys, a saltlike deposit was noticed and the skin was red and inflamed, as if a mustard plaster had been used. It was covered with blisters and very irritable. On July 13 Dr. Blanc found that the thick slime which had been blocking the urethra had now loosened, so that the urine was passed more easily and without pain.

Dr. Blanc tells of a hundred cases he treated and cured with cabbage. Among others there were cases of eczema, asthma, cystitis, sprains, cerebral inflammation, gout, inflamed eyes, headache, pleurisy, bronchitis, gangrene, toothache, burns, carbuncles, ulcers, neuralgia and phlebitis.

Which variety of cabbage is best? Many readers will be asking this question. The most effective kind is *Savoy*, but, although not quite so potent as the Savoy, the ordinary white cabbage can also be used. Red cabbage is practically useless. The Romans used to boil their cabbage for both internal and external use. Dr. Blanc and our modern naturopaths use it raw. The thickest, greenest outer leaves are most effective. They should be washed before being used.

To make a large compress, use the leaves whole. Remove the "nerves," or thick veins, and roll the leaves out so that they are flat and soft. Warm the leaves before applying them and then lay them on the place to be treated, overlapping like tiles on a roof. *For treating a small area,* cut the leaves in strips. The leaves should always be secured with a bandage. When dressing open wounds, sores or boils, the smoothest parts of the leaves should be used and care taken to see that the leaves are in contact with the whole area, otherwise some parts will be irritated more than others. The smallest crease will sometimes cause great pain.

The compresses should normally be renewed morning and evening; oftener in very bad cases. The affected area should be thoroughly washed and dried between the compresses.

As we have seen, not only surface sores and boils are affected by cabbage compresses but also deep-seated, internal processes.

Soon after the compress has been put on, there will be an increase in the suppuration. The pus may be mixed with blood and the affected part more inflamed. These signs only mean that the healing process has started. The remarkable thing is that the action of cabbage compresses is not confined to the part with which they are in contact. They also affect other diseased parts of the body, automatically attracting toxic matter which has accumulated in the tissues and is now seeking an outlet through the skin. The flow of excretion will continue until the body, and particularly the area of suppuration, has been rid of all toxic accumulations.

Fresh, green and, if possible, thick cabbage leaves should be chosen. Withered or flabby leaves are useless.

As long as the leaf is green and fresh it will be effective, however long it may remain upon the affected part. If it turns brownish, it is a sign that the excretion contains extremely strong corrosive substances.

In some cases, cabbage leaves allay pain; in others they will cause some pain in the treatment of certain troubles hitherto not painful which cannot be healed without some painful reaction.

Even in treating *intestinal infections* it is beneficial to draw the blood and toxic fluids from the irritated bowel to the exterior parts of the body. Cabbage compresses are a good febrifuge and sedative. The cabbage leaf is a sedative which never loses its effect, however long it may be used. It also acts as a disinfectant.

During my practice at Elmau, the former German Waerland sanatorium, I found the healing properties of the cabbage leaf most useful in many different cases. Our Swiss nurse sprained her foot badly, and this caused a severe effusion of blood and inflammation in the ankle, together with acute pain. Treatment with cabbage compresses for a day or two worked wonders.

An eight-year-old boy woke up one morning with a swollen, aching knee. It was too tender to be touched, and he could not stand on the leg. He was treated with compresses of cabbage leaves in bed for a couple of days, after which the swelling and pain disappeared.

We also use cabbage compresses effectively for acute migraine and sleeplessness.

Cabbage-leaf compresses are now used at all Waerland sanatoria in the various countries, where they have helped a large number of people suffering from widely different ailments.

How right Hippocrates was when he said: "Your food shall be your medicine and your medicine your food."

Now that this book is going to readers in the United States and Britain, I hope it may bring many of them new hope and new health. Perhaps also in these countries sanatoria similar to ours, which are now found in many countries in Europe, will be opened.

In my own case, after devoting some years to writing, I again feel called to work among the sick in a sanatorium. If some of my American or English readers would like to try our methods under my supervision they may write to me for specific information at the following address:

Ebba Waerland
Skärvik
Djursholm, Sweden

Glossary

Auxones / Vital substances in plants, promoting *growth.* They are found in all *living* food, fruits, roots, cereals, and green vegetables. In the fruits they are found in the peel; in root vegetables in the *whole root.* Auxones were discovered by Professor Werner Kollath (Germany). These substances are important factors in nutrition but disappear when foods are stale or have been exposed to the oxygen of the air for some time, hence *freshly ground* grains should be used for bread and kruska.

Brose / A dish made by pouring boiling water on grains—usually oatmeal. This is the name used in Scotland, the same dish being called "scalded oats" in Ireland. This dish, potatoes and sour milk, or buttermilk, formed the main diet of many rural populations in northern Europe for centuries. The fine physique of these people led Are Waerland to experiment and finally to his kruska.

Broth / "Thin or simple soup" (Webster).

Cold-pressed oils / Recent research on fats has revealed that *vegetable oils* such as wheat-germ oil, linseed oil, sunflower-seed oil, or poppy-seed oil, and some others, which have been produced simply by pressing and not exposed to heat or other complicated refining processes, are the most valuable forms of fat. This is mainly due to the fact that the *fatty acids* they contain are largely unsaturated (i.e., not fully combined with other substances or chemicals) and therefore do not increase the amount of cholesterol in the blood, whereas the acids in animal fats *are* saturated. This has been the subject of much research of late, and it has been suggested in the medical press that the excess of cholesterol from fats is probably one of the main causes of coronary thrombosis and arterio-sclerosis. Cold-pressed oils are on the market in Germany and Sweden and the United States, and to some extent in Britain. Butter, being an important source of vitamin A, should form a part of normal diet, but in moderation, being supplemented by vegetable oil. In treating certain diseases, unsaturated oil only is recommended.

Decoction / An extract obtained by boiling the substance in water. In pharmacy, *decoction* is opposed to infusion, where there is merely steeping (Webster). "If the plant is boiled in water, the strained liquor is called the *decoction* of the plant" (Arbuthnot).

Diaphoretic / inducing perspiration. Certain herbs have this property, e.g., lime-flower tea, birch-leaf tea.

Filbunke / Sour milk (bowl of). See "Recipes."

Homeopathy / The method of treating disease by drugs given in minute doses which would produce in a healthy person symptoms similar to those of the disease.

Infuse / To soak, or steep in water. The accepted use of the word nowadays is to pour *boiling* water on a substance, or herb, as in making tea, but an *infusion* is never actually boiled.

Kruska / Porridge, or brose, made from coarsely ground or whole grains, bran, and raisins. This dish was composed by Are Waerland and is an important feature of his diet system. Being very lightly cooked, it contains many valuable food elements and its bulk brings into use the now normally neglected *caecum.* On this account Sir Arthur Keith was much interested in Kruska, which Are Waerland demonstrated to him personally.

Long Milk / Milk from cows grazing in fields where *Butterwort* is abundant, when soured, becomes thick, creamy, and viscous. It is exceedingly *good* and acts as a complement to the mucus of the digestive tract. A culture can be taken during the butterwort season and made to last many months until the next season.

Rawkost / (from Swedish *rå,* "raw," and *kost,* "fare" or "food"). For the purposes of this book the term *rawkost* is used to indicate the *vegetable meal* of the normal Waerland diet, given in the "Daily Program for Health," although this meal includes one or two lightly cooked items, e.g., potatoes. The effectiveness of the reformed diet is attributable to the mainly uncooked foods.

Sauerkraut / (German: "sour cabbage"). A popular German dish of shredded cabbage "pickled" by allowing it to ferment naturally in its own juice, flavored with juniper. Only the recipe given in this book is recommended for health.

Sauna / Finnish name for the *steam baths* used in that country since ancient times. In the primitive form, still used in rural Finland, a heap of stones is heated by a fire built inside it in the bath hut. Water poured upon the hot stones creates steam. The bathers sit or lie on benches around the sides of the hut, perspiring profusely and creating a cooling "shower" by dipping birch sprays in a bucket of cold water, also beating themselves—and each other—with the sprays of birch to stimulate further the action of the skin. The final stage is a plunge in the lake or roll in the snow.

Hot, *dry* air is now thought to be more beneficial than steam. The modern *Sauna* is to be found in all the public baths and clinics providing various types of bath in Scandinavia. Elsewhere, the Turkish bath is the nearest approach to the *Sauna,* although some establishments now also have the Finnish type.

Slalom / Type of skiing involving the negotiation of difficult bends on steep slopes. International competitions held.

Sourdough / (Swedish: surdeg—"sour dough"). "A portion of fermenting dough which, when mixed with a larger quantity of dough, produces a general change in the mass and renders it light" (Webster). In olden times it was usual to save a portion of the dough, when baking, to leaven the next batch. For some conditions, this method of leavening is more suitable than using fresh yeast and is still used to make sour rye bread.

Quantities

1 liter: 1.057 U.S. liquid quarts
1 deciliter: 0.1057 U.S. liquid quarts
1 kilogram: 2.2 pounds, avoirdupois
1 gram: 0.035 ounce, avoirdupois
1 quart: 4 cups
1 tablespoon: 3 teaspoons
1 ounce, avoirdupois: 28.35 grams
1 pound, avoirdupois: 453.6 grams or approx. .45 kilograms

Note to British readers: British quarts are larger than American liquid quarts by the ratio of 12 to 10. To change American liquid quarts to British quarts, it is necessary to divide by 1.2 or to multiply by .833.

Index

Abscesses, 184-86
Acorns, decoction made from, 217
Agar-agar, 174
Air, pure, need for, 9-10
Alkaline diet, 57-58, 202
Alkaline salts, 6
Anemia, 160-63
  diet, 161-63
  treatment, 160-63
Animal protein, 4, 6
Apples, medicinal value of, 214-15
Arthritis, 47
  case histories, 52-55
  fern remedy, 225
  juniper compresses for, 212
  treatment, 55-57
Asthma, 59-66
  case histories, 63-66
  diet, 61-62
  treatment, 62
Auxones, 241

Baths, 20-21
  pine-needle, 220
  warm soda, 202-3
Bean-pod tea, 82, 88, 89-90
  recipe, 195
Birch, healing properties of, 217-19
Birch tar, 219
Birch-leaf tea, 218-19
Blackthorn, 218
Blueberries, 29
Bran, 16, 17, 24, 29
Bread for rheumatism, recipe, 195-196
Breakfast, 16-17, 27, 30
  asthmatics, 61
  cancer patients, 77
  diabetic patients, 88-89
  dropsy patients, 139
  eczema patients, 93
  gall-bladder patients, 125
  gastric-ulcer patients, 101, 102
  intestinal catarrh patients, 112
  kidney patients, 126
  liver patients, 126
  psoriasis patients, 93
  rheumatic patients, 57
Breathing, deep, 21, 189-91
Bronchitis, 60
Brose, 241
Broth, vegetable, 209

Cabbage
  compresses, 152, 181, 196-97, 235-40
  medicinal properties, 234-40
Calcium treatment for tuberculosis, 197
Camomile
  bath, 197
  compresses, 223
  medicinal properties, 222-23
  tea, 222-23
Cancer, 67-77
  case histories, 71-75
  causes, 6, 7, 68
  diet, 77
  of the lungs, 7
  treatment, 75-77
    by fasting, 45-46
Case histories
  arthritis, 52, 55
  asthma, 63-66

Case histories (*cont.*)
cancer, 71-75
diabetes, 83-85
eczema, 94-97
gall-bladder diseases, 116-19
gastric ulcers, 103-7
goitre, 174-79
gout, 50-52
headaches, 152-55
heart disorders, 167-71
intestinal disorders, 103-10
kidney diseases, 116-23
leg ulcers, 181-86
liver diseases, 116-19
migraine, 152-54
multiple sclerosis, 128-29, 132-134
paralytic diseases, 128-34
psoriasis, 94
sinusitis, 187-88
smoking, 155-57
tuberculosis, 144-48
Waerland, Ebba, 31-42
Catarrh, intestinal, 110-13
apple cure, 214
diet, 112-13
Lady's Mantle remedy, 228
treatment, 110-12
Chlorophyll, 7-8, 160-61, 163
Cholesterol, 4, 75
Cocoa, 6
Coffee, 6, 19
Colds, 60, 148
Colitis, 26, 28
Coloring matter, 6
Coltsfoot, medicinal uses, 232-33
Compresses, *see also* Poultices
cabbage, 152, 181, 196-97, 235-240
camomile, 223
juniper, 212
Condiments, 6
Cones, spruce, medicinal qualities of, 220
Constipation, 7, 158-59
causes, 56
spotted fern decoction for, 226
treatment, 158-59
Cottage (curd) cheese, recipe, 197
Crataegus, 137, 165, 224

Dandelion, medicinal uses, 231-32
Diabetes, 78-90
case histories, 83-85
diet, 88-90
treatment, 86-88
Diarrhea, 28, 29, 30
Diet, Waerland, 4, 13, 16-20
adaptations, 18-19
anemic patients, 161-63
asthmatics, 61-62
cancer patients, 77
constipated patients, 158-59
diabetic patients, 88-90
dropsy patients, 139
eczema patients, 93-94
gall-bladder patients, 124-25
gastric-ulcer patients, 19, 100-3
headache patients, 155-56
heart patients, 165-67
highly alkaline, 57-58, 202
hyperpietic patients, 163-65
impaired digestive organs and the, 26-30
insomnia patients, 157
intestinal catarrh patients, 112-113
kidney patients, 126
limited, 201-2
liver patients, 126
making change-over to, 22-30
migraine patients, 153-54
multiple sclerotic patients, 135
paralytic patients, 135
psoriasis patients, 93-94
rheumatic patients, 19, 57-58
sinusitis patients, 186-88
tubercular patients, 142-44
varicose veins and, 180
Digestive glands, 99, 111
Digestive organs, impaired, and the Waerland diet, 26-30
Digestive system, 4-5, 98-99
Dinner, 17-18, 27, 30

asthmatics, 61
cancer patients, 77
diabetic patients, 89
dropsy patients, 139
eczema patients, 93
gall-bladder patients, 125
gastric-ulcer patients, 101, 102
intestinal catarrh patients, 113
liver patients, 126
psoriasis patients, 93
rheumatic patients, 58
Drink, morning, 15-16, 24, 27, 30
asthmatics, 61
cancer patients, 77
constipated patients, 158
diabetic patients, 88
dropsy patients, 139
eczema patients, 93
"Excelsior" recipe, 199
gall-bladder patients, 125
gastric-ulcer patients, 100, 101
intestinal catarrh patients, 112
psoriasis patients, 93
rheumatic patients, 57
Dropsy, 136-41
case histories, 138-41
diet, 139
treatment, 136-41
Duodenal ulcers, *see* Ulcers
Dysentery, apple cure for, 214-15

Eczema, 91-97
case histories, 94-97
diet, 93-94
horsetail remedy, 230
treatment, 92-93
Elder, medicinal qualities, 220-21
Elderberries, 221
Elderflower tea, 221
Elimination, 13, 16-17, 23
Emotions, health and the, 11-12, 14
Enemas, 14, 19, 23-24, 28, 43
fasting and, 201
gastric-ulcer patients, 198-99
"Excelsior," recipe for, 199
Exercise, 21, 43, 162
Eye remedies, 230, 231
Eyebright, medicinal uses, 230

Fasting
on raw juices, 27, 43, 45
instructions for, 199-200
physiologically correct, 43-46
Ferns
medicinal, 224-25
spotted, 226-27
Fever
artificially induced, 148-49
willow bark remedy, 213
Flour, refined white, 7, 19
Food, *see also* Diet
animal protein, poisons produced by, 4
Fruit, 17

Gall-bladder diseases, 114
case histories, 116-19
diet, 124-25
horsetail remedy, 229
treatment, 114-16, 123-26
Gastric ulcers, *see* Ulcers
Glands, digestive, 99, 111
Glossary, 241-45
Goitre, 172-79
case histories, 174-79
diet, 173-74
medicinal fern decoction for, 225
treatment, 173-74
Gout, case history, 50-52

Hawthorn, medicinal properties, 224
Head massage, 16
Headaches, 151-57
diet, 155-56
Health
building, 3-12
daily program for, 15-21
emotions and, 11-12, 14
maintaining, 3-12
mental, 192-93
notes for, 19
rules, 13-14

Heart disorders, 28, 165-71
  case histories, 167-71
  diet, 165-67
  hawthorn remedy, 224
  treatment, 165-67
Heather, 228-29
Herbs, *see also* names of herbs, 210-40
High blood pressure, 163-65
  diet, 163-65
  treatment, 163-65
Homeopathy, defined, 242
Horsetail, medicinal uses, 229-30

Insomnia, 157-58
  camomile tea remedy, 223
  diet, 157
  treatment, 157-58
Intestinal catarrh, *see* Catarrh
Intestinal disorders, 98-113
  case histories, 107-10

Juices, raw vegetable
  fasting on, 27, 43, 45
    instructions for, 199-200
  preparation of, 205
Juniper berries, 211-12
Juniper tea, 212

Kaolin, 112
Kidney diseases, 114
  case histories, 116-23
  diet, 126
  horsetail remedy, 229
  treatment, 114-16, 123-24, 126
Kruska, 17
  defined, 243
  recipe for, 203-4
  rice, recipe for, 205-6

Lady's Mantle, medicinal properties, 228
Laxatives, 14
Leg ulcers, *see* Ulcers
Leucocytosis, digestive, 4-5
Lime, medicinal properties of, 221-222
Lime-flower tea, 221-22
Limited diet, 201-2
Linden, 222
Linseed, 16, 17, 24, 28, 29
Liver diseases, 114
  case histories, 116-19
  diet, 126
  treatment, 114-16, 123-24, 126
Long milk, 208, 243
Lunch, 17, 27, 30
  asthmatics, 61
  cancer patients, 77
  diabetic patients, 89
  dropsy patients, 139
  eczema patients, 93
  gall-bladder patients, 125
  gastric-ulcer patients, 101, 102
  intestinal catarrh patients, 113
  kidney patients, 126
  liver patients, 126
  psoriasis patients, 93
  rheumatic patients, 57-58
Lungs
  cancer of the, *see* Cancer
  tuberculosis of the, *see* Tuberculosis

Massage, head, 16
Migraine, 151-54
  case histories, 152-54
  diet, 153-54
  treatment, 151-52
Mental health, 192-93
Milk, 9, 20
  long, 208, 243
  sour, 17, 24, 28, 30
    preparation of, 207-8
Milk sugar, 17, 25
Molino, 17, 19
  recipe, 204
Morning drink, *see* Drink, morning
Multiple sclerosis, 127-35
  case histories, 128-29, 132-34
  diet, 135
  treatment, 127-34
Myasthenia gravis pseudoparalytica, 134

Nervous diseases, 11, 28
Nettles, 233-34
Nicotine, 6, 155-57

Oak bark, 216-17
Onion poultice, instructions for making, 204-5
Overacidity, 48, 56

Paralytic diseases, *see also* Multiple sclerosis
  case histories, 128-34
  diet, 135
Pine, medicinal qualities of, 219-20
Pine-needles baths, 220
Plantival, 157
Poisons, produced by animal protein food, 4
Porridge, *see also* Molino
  potato, recipe, 205
Potato porridge, 17
Poultices, *see also* Compresses
  camomile, 223
  onion, 204-5
Preservatives, artificial, 6
Protein, animal, 4, 6
Psoriasis, 91-97
  case history, 94
  diet, 93-94
  treatment, 92-93

Rawkost, 5, 13, 48, 243
Recipes
  bread for rheumatism, 195-96
  cottage cheese, 197
  decoction for gastric-ulcer patients, 100, 198
  "Excelsior," 199
  kruska, 203-4
    rice, 205-6
  molino, 204
  potato porridge, 205
  sauerkraut, 206-7
  tea
    bean-pod, 195
    birch-leaf, 219
    camomile, 222
    coltsfoot, 232
    dandelion, 232
    elderflower, 221
    hawthorn, 224
    lime-flower, 221-22
    nettle, 233-34
    yarrow, 227-28
Respiratory diseases, *see also* Tuberculosis
Rheumatism, 47-49
  bread for, recipe, 195-96
  causes, 6, 56
  dandelion remedy, 232
  diet, 19, 57-58
  heather decoction for, 228
  medicinal fern remedy, 225-26
  treatment, 55-57
  willow bark remedy, 213
Rice kruska, recipe for, 205-6
Rose hips, as source of vitamin C, 216
Rusks, 29

Salicylic acid, 213
Salizin, 213
Salt, commercial, 6, 19, 56
Sauerkraut, 24-25, 243-44
  recipe, 206-7
Sauna, 14, 43, 244
Sclerosis, *see* Multiple sclerosis
Silicic acid, 229, 230
Sinusitis, 186-88
  case history, 187-88
  diet, 186-88
  treatment, 186-87
Skin, care of, 16
Sleeplessness, *see* Insomnia
Smoking, 6-7, 155-57
Soda baths, warm, 202-3
Sodium chloride, 6
Soil, health of the, 8-9
Sour milk, 17, 24, 28, 30
  preparation of, 207-8
Sourdough, 207, 244-45
Soya beans, sprouted, 208
Spices, 6
Spiritual life, 194

Sprouted soya beans, 208
Sprouted wheat, 208
Spruce, medicinal qualities of, 219-220
Stinging nettle, 233-34
Stomach disorders, 98-113
Sugar
  refined, 6
  white, 6
Sugar cane, 6
Supper, *see* Dinner

Tannin, 216
Tapeworms, remedy for, 225
Tea, 6, 19
  bean-pod, 82, 88, 89-90
    recipe, 195
  birch-leaf, 218-19
  camomile, 222-23
  coltsfoot, 232-33
  dandelion, 231-32
  elderflower, 221
  hawthorn, 224
  juniper, 212
  Lady's Mantle, 228
  lime-flower, 221-22
  nettle, 233-34
  rose-hip, 216
  willow bark, 213
  yarrow, 227-28
Tilia, 221-22
Tobacco, 6-7, 19, 155-57
Tuberculosis, 28, 46, 142-48
  case histories, 144-48
  diet, 142-44
  horsetail remedy, 229
  treatment, 142-48
    calcium, 197

Ulcers
  gastric, 99
    case histories, 103-7
    decoction for (recipe), 100, 198
    diet, 19, 100-3
    enemas and, 198-99
  leg, 181-86
    cabbage compresses for, 235
    case histories, 181-86
    horsetail remedy, 229-30

Varicose veins, 180-81
  diet, 180
  treatment, 180-81
Vegetable broth, 209
Vegetable juices, *see* Juices, raw vegetable
Vitamin C, rose hips as source of, 216

Waerland, Ebba, case history, 31-42
Walk, morning, 16
Warm soda baths, instructions for, 202-3
Water, drinking, 15-16
Wheat, sprouted, 208-9
Willow bark, 213-14

Yarrow, medicinal properties, 227-228
Yogurt, 17, 24, 209

9780718891299

ND - #0030 - 230726 - C0 - 216/138/15 - PB - 9780718891299 - Gloss Lamination